Prostate cancer

A NON-SURGICAL PERSPECTIVE

Prostate cancer
A NON-SURGICAL PERSPECTIVE

Kent Wallner, M.D.

SmartMedicine Press
Canaan, New York

First Edition

Library of Congress Catalog Card Number: 95-90687
ISBN: 0-9648991-0-8

Published by SmartMedicine Press, Canaan, New York
Printed by Marrakech Express, Tarpon Springs, Florida
Marketing consultant: Greg Lawrence
Cover design by Deborah Rust

Distributor to the trade: Publishers Distribution Service
                            6893 Sullivan Road
                            Grawn, Michigan 49637
                            (616) 276-5196

Dedicated to my wife, Kathryn,
whose love, support and patience
helped make this possible.

Acknowledgements

The following people share credit for this book. Each has contributed by editing the work, or by suggesting ways to best present the material.

Joel Azerrad
Daniel Clarke, M.D.
Guido Dalbagni, M.D.
Kathryn Elliott, M.D.
Lindsay Elliott
Louis Harrison, M.D.
Chris Jacobs
Eric Klein, M.D.
Ron Koster
Greg Lawrence
David Nanus, M.D.
Kenneth Russell, M.D.
Lewis E. Wallner, Sr.

Contents

Illustrations

Caution:

This book is intended to supplement, but not replace, the advice of qualified physicians. It is imperative that you seek advice from qualified physicians regarding your particular situation.

1

Why this book

Treatment of prostate cancer is one of the most controversial areas in medicine. A major component of this controversy is determining whether treatment is necessary. Another area of dispute is determining which treatment is best when treatment is necessary. Considerable disagreement exists among doctors as to the answers to these questions. Ultimately, the decision to accept treatment is up to the patient. A decision about treatment for such a complex disease is a difficult one to make, especially when one will probably get conflicting advice from different specialists.

It is common to get conflicting advice because like everyone else, doctors have biases. They tend to recommend what they know how to do. Surgeons tend to recommend surgery; radiation oncologists tend to recommend radiation. Both types of doctors usually recommend doing *something*.

While many men seek second opinions, many others do not. Patients may not seek other opinions because of their willingness to go along with the recommendation of the first doctor. However, with a disease whose treatment is as controversial as that for prostate cancer, you should know your treatment options. I am trained as a radiation doctor and have worked primarily with prostate cancer patients since 1987. I have extensive experience in patient care, research and education regarding external radiation and implant radiation. I wrote this book to give men and their loved ones a chance to read the perspective of a non-surgeon. This book will give you some additional guidance through a potentially bewildering maze of conflicting viewpoints. It can serve as a "second opinion."

Although the medical intricacies of the field of prostate cancer may be beyond what one could master without formal training, many of the issues to consider when choosing treatment are judgment calls. They require familiarity with general concepts, not with detailed medical procedures and statistics. These concepts, along with some current medical knowledge, are summarized in the pages ahead.

2

What is prostate cancer

Prostate cancer is the most common cancer of American men. It is second only to lung cancer as the most common cause of cancer death in men. It is diagnosed much more frequently since 1988, when screening by a new blood test (PSA) was introduced.

The prostate

The prostate is about the size of a walnut in younger men, and the size of a chicken egg in older men. It sits just below the bladder (*Figure 2a*).

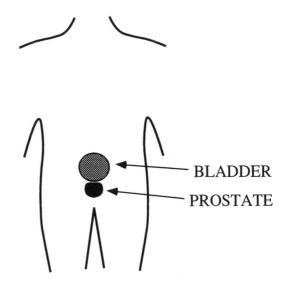

Figure 2a. Front view of the bladder and prostate.

The urine passage (urethra) leads from the bladder through the prostate on its way to the penis (*Figure 2b*).

The prostate's main function is to produce part of the ejaculate fluid, which empties into the urethra at the

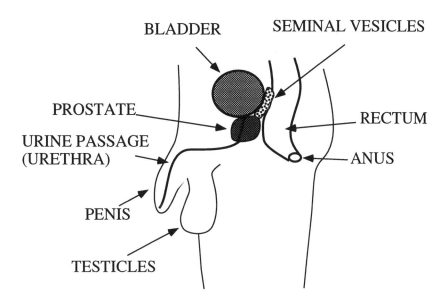

Figure 2b. Side view of the male pelvis. The prostate sits just in front of the rectum. The back of the prostate can be felt by placing a finger into the rectum (digital rectum exam).

time of orgasm. This fluid helps carry sperm through the penis at the time of ejaculation.

Seminal vesicles are two sack-like structures attached to the back of the prostate. These vesicles produce extra fluid that passes through the prostate during ejaculation.

Cancer

The prostate is composed of hundreds of small passages lined with cells that produce the ejaculate fluid. These lining cells normally reproduce slowly. As some cells get older and die, they are replaced by younger cells underneath. Normally, the cells reproduce just often enough to replace the dying cells. With cancer, some cells go haywire and start to reproduce uncontrollably. Consequently, there is a build-up of cells, all growing out of control. Such cells are called cancer cells. This pile-up of cancer cells in the prostate causes a lump. The medical term for lump is "tumor." Things besides cancer can cause a lump or tumor in the body, including infection, bruising, etc. While technically the word tumor does not necessarily mean a cancerous lump, "tumor" is commonly used as a synonym for cancer.

A cancer growing inside the prostate usually causes no symptoms because it grows slowly, and essentially incorporates itself within the normal tissue. Men with prostate cancer often have frequent urination, slow urine stream and get up once or more during the night to urinate (nocturia), but these symptoms usually reflect overgrowth of normal prostate tissue that commonly occurs with aging (benign prostatic hypertrophy).

Prostate cancer is common

Prostate cancer is very common and becomes more prevalent as men get older. This cancer is present in approximately 15% of men at age 55, 30% of men at age 65, and in 45% of men at age 75 (*Figure 2c*).

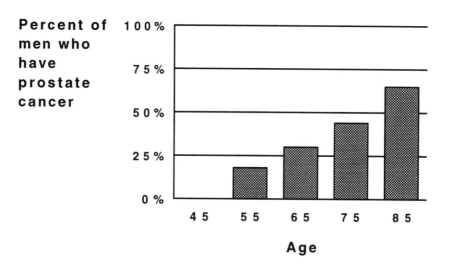

Figure 2c. The prevalence of prostate cancer increases dramatically in men above age 55.

The cause of prostate cancer is largely unknown. Researchers have found that people who have relatives with prostate cancer are more likely to get this cancer. However, heredity is only a small part of the cause. A high fat diet may increase the chance of getting prostate cancer.

While almost half of older men have cancer within the prostate, the good news is that only about 6% of these men will die from it. In fact, only a small fraction of cancers ever grow large enough to spread beyond the prostate. What makes cancer grow quickly in some men and not in others is unknown.

Spread of cancer through the prostate capsule

Cancer cells have the potential to spread to other parts of the body. Whatever changes occurred to cause cancer cells to reproduce uncontrollably, also frees them of their natural tendency to stay in their proper place within the prostate.

When a prostate cancer first starts, it is confined to the prostate. This is what is known as "early stage prostate cancer." It is at this early stage that the cancer is potentially curable, either by surgically removing the prostate, or by radiating the prostate.

However, by the time cancers are diagnosed, only about half of them are still confined to the prostate.

As a cancer enlarges, it grows towards the edge of the prostate. Given enough time, it can grow through the outer edge of the prostate called the "capsule." This is known as "extra capsular extension." It is a very important concept, because once extra capsular extension occurs, it is less likely that a man can be cured.

Cancer can also escape the prostate by growing up along the seminal vesicles where the vesicles attach at the back of the prostate. Cancer growth into the seminal vesicles makes it less likely that a man can be cured.

Spread of cancer to other areas of the body

Cancer can also escape from the prostate by getting into a blood or lymph vessel. Lymph channels form a drainage system throughout the body to drain excess fluid to the bloodstream. Along these channels are lymph nodes, which serve as traps that stop cancer cells traveling in the lymph fluid. Cancer cells can move into lymph vessels or blood vessels that run through the prostate. Once cancer cells get inside a vessel, they may be carried away to other parts of the body to form a new area of cancer. A cancer that spreads through the blood or lymph system is said to "metastasize." The new areas of cancer growth are termed "metastases." Metastases are still considered to be prostate cancer because the cells originated in the prostate. Metastases most frequently develop in the lymph nodes or the bones, usually the spine.

Types of doctors that specialize in prostate cancer

The treatment of prostate cancer is divided into several medical specialties, each of which approach the issue from different perspectives.

Urologists are surgeons who spend one year after medical school studying general surgery. They spend three additional years studying the surgical care of the urinary tract and sexual organs.

Radiation oncologists are doctors who spend one year after medical school studying general medical care and three additional years studying the use of radiation for all types of cancer.

Medical oncologists are doctors who spend two years after medical school studying general internal medicine and then two additional years studying the use of chemotherapy and hormonal therapy for cancer.

The division between specialists is not always clear. Radiation implants of the prostate, for instance, are sometimes performed by urologists with little input from a radiation oncologist. Similarly, both urologists and radiation oncologists often prescribe hormonal therapy which might otherwise be prescribed by a medical oncologist.

3

The work-up

Once you are diagnosed with prostate cancer, several tests are done to help define the extent of the disease. "Work-up" is the medical term for a series of tests used to determine how advanced a cancer is. The results of these tests are used to determine the type of treatment most appropriate for your particular cancer.

Digital rectal exam (DRE)

The rectal exam is the simplest way to estimate how advanced a cancer is. Most cancers are located in the back portion of the prostate. If a cancer is large enough, it can be felt by placing a finger (digit) inside the rectum against the prostate. Cancers that have grown against the edge of the prostate can be felt as a lump. It may be possible to tell, by the size and shape of the lump, whether a cancer has grown through the prostate capsule.

Unfortunately, the rectal exam is not particularly accurate. Many cancers do not grow in such a way that they protrude against the back of the prostate. If they extend to the front of the prostate they cannot be felt through the rectum. Additionally, there is often disagreement among doctors as to how a particular cancer feels. Because of its subjective nature, the rectal exam provides only an estimation of how advanced a cancer really is. In fact, approximately one half of cancers that feel as though they are confined to the prostate will have grown outside of the prostate.

PSA (prostate specific antigen)

PSA is a protein produced by the cells lining the internal prostatic channels. A small amount of PSA normally leaks into blood vessels inside the prostate and flows into the bloodstream. The amount of PSA in the blood can be measured by a simple laboratory test.

Prostate cancers usually produce extra PSA which can be detected in the bloodstream. PSA is also produced by prostate cancer cells that have metastasized to other parts of the body.

Several different companies sell PSA tests. Most have a normal range of 0 to 4. A PSA greater than 4 is considered abnormal. For clarity, all PSA values in this book are stated with a normal range of 0-4 ng/ml. From here on, the units of measure (ng/ml) will not be included.

Several conditions, besides prostate cancer, can cause an elevation of the PSA. The most common is prostatic enlargement that commonly occurs with aging. The medical term for non-cancerous enlargement is benign prostatic hypertrophy (BPH). BPH will not generally elevate the PSA above 10. Infection or biopsy of the prostate can also temporarily elevate the PSA. A rectal examination will not usually cause an increase in the PSA.

An elevated PSA level gives a rough approximation of the size of a cancer. The higher the PSA, the larger the cancer and the greater the chance that it has already grown through the prostate capsule (*Figure 3a*).

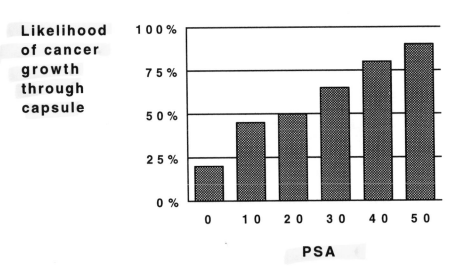

Figure 3a. The likelihood that cancer has grown through the prostate capsule, versus PSA.

While there is a correlation between cancer size and the PSA, the relation is only approximate. Some cancers can grow very large but still not cause a significant elevation of the PSA. It is important to remember that the description of all cancer tests are given in terms of probabilities. Some men with a very high PSA value still have small, curable cancers. Conversely, some men with a low PSA have more advanced cancers. Despite the exceptions to the rule, the PSA is a valuable tool.

Gleason score

Not all prostate cancers behave the same. They exhibit a range of aggressiveness, from slow-growing to fast-growing. When a biopsy is taken of the prostate, the tissue is soaked in a preservative solution, cut into thin slices, and examined under a microscope. Some cancers appear more aggressive, or fast-growing, than others. Cancers that look similar to normal prostatic tissue are called "well differentiated," while those that look very abnormal are termed "poorly differentiated." Cancers that appear somewhere in between are termed "moderately differentiated."

The Gleason score quantifies how aggressive (fast-growing) a cancer appears. The score increases from 2 to 10, with 2 being the slowest growing cancers and 10 the more aggressive (*Figure 3b*). The higher the Gleason number, the more likely a cancer is fast-growing, and has already grown through the capsule of the prostate or metastasized (*Figure 3c*).

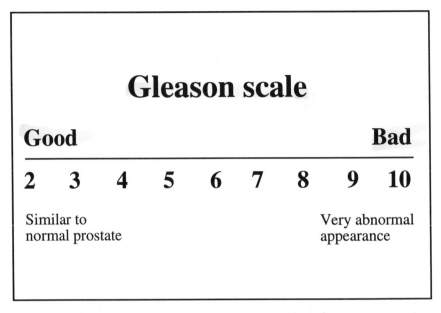

Figure 3b. The Gleason score quantifies how aggressive a cancer appears under a microscope, on a scale of 2-10.

Like the PSA, the Gleason score provides only an approximation of the aggressiveness of a cancer. Cancers are often heterogeneous. Some parts of a cancer may look more aggressive than other parts, depending on which part is sampled by the biopsy needle. By chance, then, the Gleason number might give a false idea of a cancer's aggressiveness. Some men with a high Gleason score may have small, curable cancers. Conversely, some men with a low score may have more advanced cancers. Despite room for

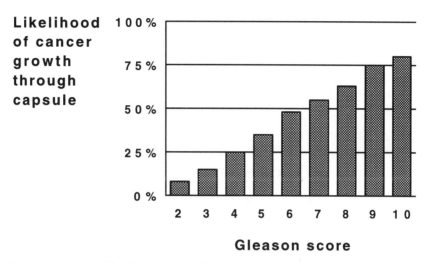

Figure 3c. The likelihood that cancer has grown through the prostate capsule, versus the Gleason score.

error in its use, the Gleason score provides a good idea of the aggressive nature of a cancer.

Other scales besides the Gleason have been devised. However, the Gleason scale is the most widely used. In some biopsy samples, it is difficult to assign a Gleason number, in which case the cancer is simply described as well differentiated, moderately differentiated or poorly differentiated.

Bone scan

The most common place for prostate cancer to metastasize is the bones. Consequently, an important part of the work-up is to check for abnormalities of the bones, with a bone scan.

A bone scan is performed by injecting a small amount of radioactive dye (technetium) into a patient's arm vein. The dye circulates through the bloodstream and is absorbed by irritated areas in the bone. An image of the skeleton is obtained by lying under a radioactive detection camera for several minutes. Irritation of the bone, whatever the cause, shows up as a dark spot on the image (*Figure 3d*).

Irritation of the bone due to a prior injury or to arthritis is the most common cause of an abnormality on a bone scan. Irritation can also be caused by cancer that has metastasized to the bone.

An abnormal finding on a bone scan is often not specific, in that it is not certain whether it is due to cancer or arthritis, or some other cause. In such cases, plain x-rays or a CT scan (see below) may be done of the area in question to clarify the cause of an abnormality.

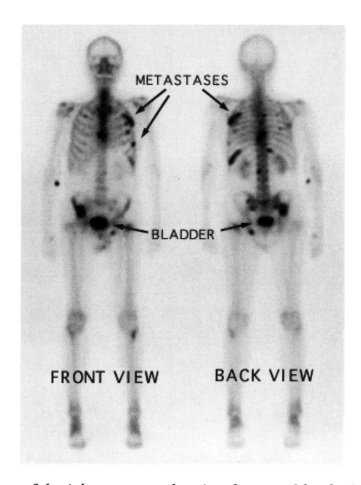

Figure 3d. A bone scan, showing front and back view of the skeleton. Arrows point to metastases and to the bladder, which shows up well because much of the radioactive dye is eliminated via the urine.

The likelihood of finding metastases on a bone scan relates to the PSA value. With a PSA below 20, the likelihood of finding cancer on a scan is less than 1% (1 in 100). With a PSA of 100, the likelihood of detecting cancer is approximately 50% (*Figure 3e*).

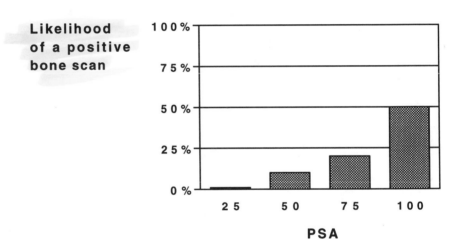

Likelihood of a positive bone scan

PSA

Figure 3e. The likelihood of a positive bone scan increases for men who have a higher PSA at the time of diagnosis.

Ultrasound

Another test used to determine the extent of a prostate cancer is the ultrasound. Sound waves are used to visualize the prostate. The sound waves are generated by a round probe placed inside the rectum. Reflections of the sound waves from the prostate generate an image of the prostate on a screen. Cancer within the prostate generally appears as a dark spot (*Figure 3f*).

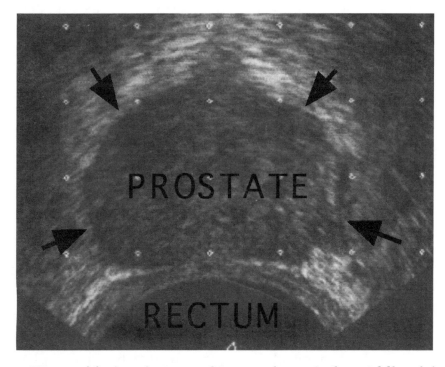

Figure 3f. An ultrasound image through the middle of the prostate. Note that the picture is quite fuzzy. It is good for directing biopsies of the prostate, but not as good as MRI for seeing cancers (Courtesy of Michael Dattoli, M.D.).

Ultrasound may identify areas where a cancer has grown through the prostate capsule. However, ultrasound is not very accurate in determining these areas. Approximately 50% of men in whom ultrasound does not show penetration of the capsule will, in fact, have an area of penetration. Areas of cancer growth through the capsule are often simply too small to be seen. Also, other abnormalities of the prostate, including infections, can be mistaken for cancer.

CT scan

CT scans (also called "CAT scans") are computer-reconstructed x-rays that give a cross-sectional view of the body. A CT scan through the pelvis shows the outline of the prostate (*Figure 3g*).

These scans are used primarily to look for enlarged lymph nodes around the prostate. Although CT scans are good for determining the size and shape of the prostate, they are not accurate at visualizing cancers within the prostate.

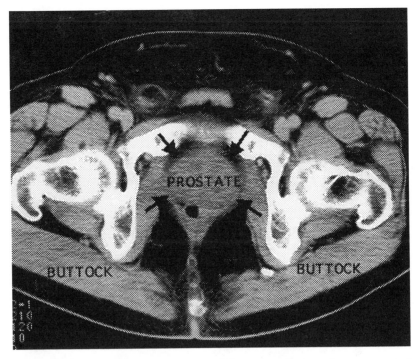

Figure 3g. Example of a CT scan through a normal prostate. Although the outline of the prostate can be seen, the CT scan does not give a detailed enough image of the prostate to see small cancers (Courtesy of Lawrence H. Schwartz, M.D.).

MRI

Another test that is used to look for evidence of cancer having grown outside of the prostate is magnetic resonance imaging (MRI). It relies on a strong magnet to align hydrogen protons within the body. Energy in the form of a radiofrequency wave is emitted from an antenna within the MRI machine, making the protons go out of alignment. As they return to their baseline state, energy is given off, and is measured by the MRI machine and converted into an image (*Figure 3h*).

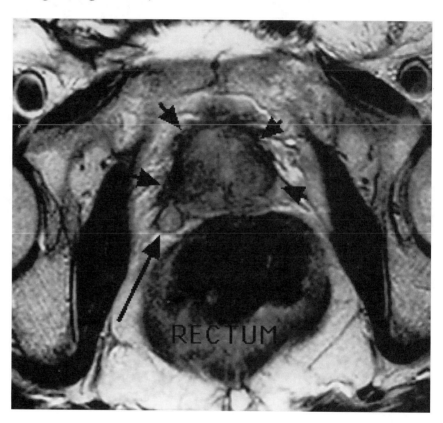

Figure 3h. On an MRI scan, one can see the outline of the prostate (short arrows). The cancer itself is growing outside of the prostate (long arrow) (Courtesy of Lawrence H. Schwartz, M.D.).

MRI is primarily used to identify cancer that has grown through the prostate capsule. MRI scans are more accurate than CT scans or ultrasound in detecting capsular penetration.

However, 30% of men in whom MRI does not show penetration of the capsule will still have some penetration, too small to be detected.

Recently, an accessory MRI tool (a rectal coil) has become widely available. Inserted in the rectum during the scan, it allows sharper pictures of the prostate. A rectal coil should be used to get optimal images of the prostate.

Lymph nodes

One of the first areas that cancer spreads to is the lymph nodes around the prostate. Once cancer has spread to the lymph nodes, there is little chance of cure with available treatment. Treatment options would include surgical removal of the lymph nodes, radiation, or hormonal treatment. However, in these cases, probably the best "treatment" is no treatment, although there is still considerable debate in this regard.

CT scans or MRI scans can show enlarged lymph nodes that are likely to be cancerous. However, lymph nodes containing cancer are usually not large enough to show up on scans. The only way to be sure whether or not there is cancer present in these nodes is to surgically remove them and examine them under a microscope. Because local treatment to the prostate is not advised if cancer has spread to the lymph nodes, it has been argued that the lymph nodes should be removed ("sampled") before a patient undergoes surgery or radiation.

Until the late 1980s, sampling of lymph nodes around the prostate required an operation through the lower abdomen. More recently, limited surgery, using thin tubes (laparoscopes) to see and work through, has been devised. Laparoscopic removal of lymph nodes around the prostate is done through five small incisions in the lower abdomen. This surgery entails less risk of complications and eliminates the need for a long hospitalization. Patients can usually go home the next day.

Routine lymph node sampling is controversial. Men with low PSAs and low Gleason scores are unlikely to have cancer in the lymph nodes. Men with PSAs below 10 and Gleason scores of 6 or less have a 10%

or lower chance of having cancer in their lymph nodes. For these men, it is generally agreed that the low probability of finding cancer in the nodes does not warrant their undergoing a laparoscopy.

For men with PSA greater than 10, a Gleason score of 7 or more, or Stage C cancer (see below), the likelihood of having cancer in the lymph nodes is higher. A stronger argument can be made to do a lymph node sampling for such patients, because if their lymph nodes contain cancer, they would avoid having radiation or prostatectomy. The argument against doing a lymph node sampling is that it requires a surgical procedure, and there may be more side effects from the lymph node sampling than from the treatment itself. This debate over whether on not to undergo an operation solely to look at the lymph nodes has raged for decades.

Staging

Using the information from the studies described above, a cancer is assigned a letter from A to D. This is called assigning a "Stage."

A newer staging system has been introduced that divides cancers into stages, called T1, T2, T3 or T4.

The T system is comparable to the A through D system, except that it subdivides the stages in more detail.

Stage A cancers (T1) are not large enough to be felt by rectal examination. They are found incidentally after a TURP (surgical removal of the central portion of their prostate) or by an elevated PSA reading that leads to a biopsy.

Stage B cancers (T2) can be felt by rectal exam, but are still small enough to feel as though they are confined to the prostate capsule.

Stage C cancers (T3) are larger tumors that can be felt by rectal exam and feel as though they have grown through the capsule of the prostate.

Stage D cancers are those which have already metastasized. They may have metastasized only to the lymph nodes near the prostate (Stage D1), or further, to the bones (Stage D2).

The cancer stage indicates the likelihood of cure. There are a variety of treatments for each stage, although there is disagreement among physicians as to what precisely is the best treatment for each stage (*Figure 3i*).

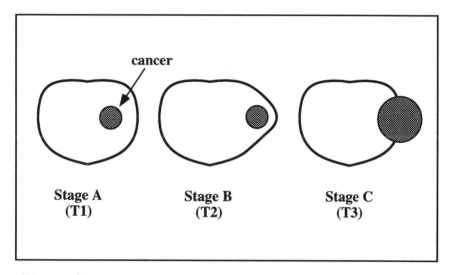

cancer

Stage A
(T1)

Stage B
(T2)

Stage C
(T3)

Figure 3i. Prostate cancers are staged based on how large the tumor feels on digital rectal examination.

Is there a hurry to make a decision?

Once a man is diagnosed with prostate cancer, the question may arise, "How long can I safely wait to decide what treatment is best?" Several weeks are often needed to schedule and go through the "work-up." Patients may become concerned that time spent getting their tests and meeting with one or more doctors will allow the cancer too much time to grow. This is not the case. Prostate cancers are usually slow-growing, and by the time a cancer is detected it has probably already been present several years. Although a diagnosis of cancer is alarming, patients have time to investigate and consider the options.

It is impossible to say just how much time one can safely wait before making a decision. It is not wise to waste time unnecessarily. However, judging from the slow rise in PSA readings over time, taking a month or so to explore one's treatment options is highly unlikely to decrease one's chance of being cured.

4

To treat or not to treat

Most men with prostate cancer will not die from it

Prostate cancer is the most common type of cancer in men. As the second leading cause of cancer deaths in men, it accounts for 3-5% of American male deaths. As men get older, it becomes even more common. By age 80, at least 50% of men will have cancer in their prostate. Although most men will develop cancer within their prostate, only a small percent of cancers grow large enough to ever be detected. In other words, most men do not live long enough to die of their prostate cancer.

A number of studies have been done in which large numbers of men with prostate cancer were followed carefully by their doctors without being treated. The studies all show that the likelihood of dying from prostate cancer, if it is diagnosed at an early stage, is small, in the first few years after diagnosis. The risk of dying from the cancer within five years of diagnosis is only about one or two out of 100. The risk of dying from the cancer stays low for the first 10 years after diagnosis. At 10 years, about 10% of men with cancer diagnosed at Stage A or B will have died from their cancer. At fifteen years after diagnosis, the likelihood of dying from prostate cancer rises to about 25% (*Figure 4a*).

Because of the low risk of dying from Stage A or B prostate cancer within 10 years of diagnosis, men with other serious health problems probably do not need treatment. For men with other serious medical conditions, treating Stage A or B cancer should be considered in light of one's life expectancy. A 60-year-old man has an average life expectancy of 20 more years. He should choose treatment for his prostate cancer because he will probably live long

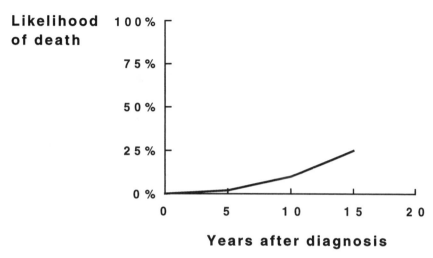

Figure 4a. The likelihood of death from untreated, Stage A or B prostate cancer.

enough to die of his prostate cancer if it is left untreated. Conversely, an 80-year-old man has an average life expectancy of eight years and is less likely to be threatened by a Stage A or B prostate cancer before dying from other causes (*Figure 4b*).

While death from Stage A or B prostate cancer within 10 years of diagnosis is unlikely, there is a risk of developing metastases. Like the risk of dying from untreated prostate cancer, the probability of developing metastases in the short term is low. The chances

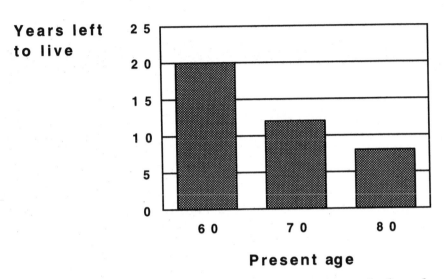

Figure 4b. Approximate life expectancy at each decade. On average, a 70 year old man has 12 more years to live.

of developing metastases within 5 years of diagnosis is about 20%, or one in five. But at 15 years, the likelihood increases to 60% (*Figure 4c*).

Developing metastases from untreated prostate cancer is more likely than the chance of dying from the cancer, because men can live with metastatic prostate cancer for many years. Although development of metastatic prostate cancer is not synonymous with death, metastatic cancer in the bones can cause pain and lead to a diminished quality of life.

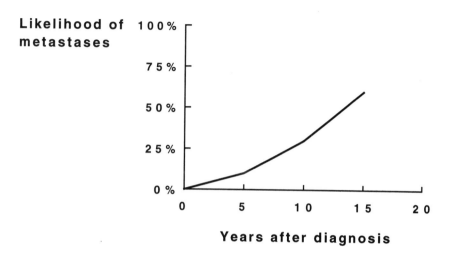

Figure 4c . The likelihood of metastases after diagnosis of Stage A or B prostate cancer, left untreated.

The decision of whether or not to be treated for prostate cancer may be made more logically if the Gleason score and PSA are considered. Cancers with a higher Gleason score are more likely to metastasize sooner rather than later. In general, cancers with a Gleason score of 7 or above tend to be faster growing, and therefore, more serious consideration should be given to their treatment. Similarly, a higher PSA usually indicates a larger cancer that should be treated sooner rather than later.

Watchful waiting

The slow-growing nature of many prostate cancers has led to growing interest in postponing treatment until some evidence reveals that the cancer is actually growing. This concept has been called "watchful waiting." It is called watchful waiting because patients are monitored by rectal examination and PSA every four months. If the rectal exam or the PSA show that the cancer is growing, treatment is almost certainly needed. The hope, of course, is that if a rise in the PSA occurs, it will not be too late for cure with either surgery or radiation.

There is some variability in the PSA from day to day and from one laboratory to another, so that it is important to get a series of PSA values over one year or longer, before deciding whether or not there is an upward trend of the PSA.

Is is unclear just how safe the policy of watchful waiting is. The question remains as to how reliable the PSA or changes in the digital rectal exam are in detecting growth. It is critical to catch the cancer before it spreads outside of the prostate. Because more and more men are choosing "watchful waiting." substantial data regarding the safety of this choice should be available in coming years.

In summary

The advocates for treatment of prostate cancer assert that the best time to eradicate a cancer is when it is smallest and least likely to have spread outside of the prostate. Those who argue against treatment stress the fact that treatment is often not needed due to the slow growing nature of most prostate cancers. In addition, all forms of treatment have the potential for complications which can adversely affect your quality of life.

In general, men under 70 are advised to seek treatment because they will probably live long enough for their cancer to grow and become life-threatening. Men over 70 should consider watchful waiting, because they are less likely to live long enough to be threatened by their cancer. These are only rough guidelines, and patients should temper these by considering their general state of health. For example, some 60-year-olds have serious heart conditions, making it unlikely that they will live long enough to be threatened by their prostate cancer. Conversely, some 80-year-olds are in excellent health and therefore should be treated.

5

The definition of cure

Remission versus cure

Being cured of prostate cancer means that a patient's entire cancer has been eradicated, permanently. The definition is simple enough. In practice, however, determining who is cured is not a simple matter.

Before the introduction of PSA monitoring, the only way to know if cancer was still present was to see if it could be felt by rectal examination, if it appeared on repeated biopsies, or if metastases showed up on a bone scan. When residual cancer was too small to be detected by a rectal exam or bone scan, a patient was erroneously considered to be cured. Someone whose cancer has shrunk down after treatment and is too small to be detected is said to be "in remission." Being in remission, however, is not the same as a cure. Patients who are in remission may show a recurrence of their cancer in the future.

Falsely high cure rates, before PSA

Before PSA testing was introduced, the chance of being cured of Stage A or B cancer by prostatectomy or radiation was thought to be 90% or more. This cure rate was falsely high as not all men were followed long enough to know if they were truly cured.

Prostate cancer is generally slow-growing, and many men whose cancer is in remission after treatment will die of other causes before their cancer has time to regrow. Those men were counted as cured even though they had simply not lived long enough to manifest signs of persistent cancer. Before PSA, it was necessary to wait 10 to 15 years after radiation or surgery to get a good idea of how many men were really cured.

When the PSA test was introduced in the 1980s it became possible to detect residual prostate cancer much sooner following treatment than was previously possible.

Shortly after surgery or radiation, a patient's cancer is usually in remission because his PSA has become undetectable or has decreased to very low levels. However, after several years, some patients will have a rise in their PSA if residual cancer is present. A detectable rise in the PSA usually means that residual cancer is present and that it is growing. Most men who have residual cancer will develop a rising PSA within five years of treatment. Those men without rising PSA after five years are probably cured. This can be shown by graphing the percentage of men with a rising PSA versus the number of years since treatment (*Figure 5a*).

One can get a rough idea of the cure rates by looking at the percentage of men without a rising PSA in the first five years after treatment. As time goes on, some additional men will have a rising PSA many years after treatment. Their cancers are very slow-growing, and they require longer for residual cancer to be detected. The ultimate cure rate, regardless of the type of treatment, may take many years to determine.

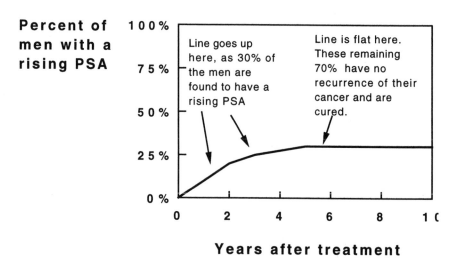

Figure 5 a. Idealized graph of cancer recurrence after treatment. In this example, 30% of men had residual cancer (rising PSA), detected within 5 years after treatment. The remaining 70% of the patients were cured, evidenced by flattening of the line after 5 years.

PSA results have shocked the medical world

PSA results showed that cure rates are lower than was previously reported. This finding shocked most physicians. A reappraisal of the treatment options ensued, as well as renewed interest in basic scientific research. The goal is to look for better ways to treat prostate cancer. Renewed interest in implant treatment for delivery of radiation, and in the use of higher doses of external radiation using computer-assisted high-precision radiation resulted from the realization that prostate cancer cure rates are lower than was previously believed.

The treatment options

The remainder of this book will review in detail the three major forms of treatment for prostate cancer: surgery (prostatectomy), and two forms of radiation (external and implants). Some information about cryotherapy, the newest type of treatment, is included. Less conventional treatments, including shark cartilage, and dietary therapy are not discussed because little or no data exists to support their use over more conventional treatments. However, one or more alternative treatment forms may someday supplant the more conventional forms.

6

Surgery

Surgery has long been held by most doctors as the most effective treatment for Stage A or B prostate cancer. Whether surgery truly is more effective than radiation is still a subject of hot debate. Good results in past reports may be due to subtle ways in which patients were chosen for surgery, as opposed to radiation. Some of these issues will be addressed later.

What is a prostatectomy

A prostatectomy is the removal of the prostate, the seminal vesicles, and the lymph nodes around the prostate. The urine passage (urethra) is then reconnected between the bladder and that portion of the urethra beyond the prostate. The operation is usually done through an incision in the central lower abdomen. The lymph nodes within the pelvis are routinely removed first, and looked at under a microscope. If cancer is seen in the lymph nodes, the operation is stopped because once cancer has spread there, it is considered incurable.

A prostatectomy takes from two to four hours to perform. On average, patients lose about 1 to 2 units of blood (1 to 2 pints) during the operation. Men are encouraged to donate their own blood in the 4 weeks preceding the operation.

Following a prostatectomy, patients remain hospitalized from 4 to 10 days. They are encouraged to start walking several hours after the operation. A catheter (a 1/4 inch thick, flexible tube) is left in the penis during the recovery period, since patients have little urine control for several weeks following the operation.

The catheter is removed two to four weeks after the procedure.

Who is eligible?

A prostatectomy is a big operation. Because of the general stress on the body, most surgeons are reluctant to do the operation on men older than 70. Younger men with serious heart conditions or other serious medical problems are usually discouraged from having the operation due to their higher risk of complications.

Men with Stage A or B cancers are most likely to have cancer confined to the prostate and therefore curable by a prostatectomy. Most surgeons will only operate on men with Stage A or B cancers. A few surgeons advocate operating on men with Stage C cancers, but only about 10% of these patients will have cancer confined to the prostate. Men with Stage C cancers are usually treated with radiation and/or hormonal therapy.

Complications of surgery

GENERAL RISKS OF AN OPERATION

Some of the complications of a prostatectomy are the same as those that accompany any big operation. These include death associated with anesthesia, formation of blood clots in the legs or lungs, or pneumonia. Fortunately, each of these complications should occur in less than 1% of patients. There is also a 1% risk of rectal damage.

URINE INCONTINENCE

When a man's prostate is removed, the urine passage within the prostate is also removed and the remaining ends are reconnected. This trauma to the passage causes temporary incontinence (involuntary urine leakage) in all men. Most patients regain their urine control within several weeks to months of the operation. However, some are left with permanent incontinence.

A wide range of incontinence severity exists following a prostatectomy. Some patients are left with only slight control problems where they may occasionally lose a few drops of urine when lifting heavy objects or coughing ("stress incontinence"). Other men are left with very little control over their urine flow, and have to wear absorbent pads in their underwear.

Depending on which medical research report one reads, the likelihood that a patient will experience incontinence can vary from 2 to 65%. This surprisingly large range of numbers partly reflects the differences in definitions doctors use to describe "incontinence." If a patient has only slight urine leakage, some doctors report that the patient is not incontinent. Other doctors consider any urine leakage, at any time, to be incontinence. A realistic estimate of the risk of some incontinence is probably around 10%, in very good surgical hands.

SEXUAL POTENCY

Impotence refers to the inability to have an erection, while the desire for sex remains unchanged. Like urinary incontinence, there is a wide range in the severity of impotence following a prostatectomy. Some patients are left with only a slight decreased firmness of their erections; other patients are left unable to have erections. However, having said that, prostate cancer patients should know that effective methods of restoring erections are available (see Chapter 11).

Until the 1980s, nearly all patients undergoing prostatectomy were left permanently impotent. In the early 1980s, Dr. Patrick Walsh of Johns Hopkins Hospital devised a technique to remove the prostate while leaving intact the nerves that control erections. To perform this "nerve-sparing" operation, the nerves are identified along the back of the prostate and care is taken not to injure them. Because these nerves are small and so close to the prostate, the chance of removing a man's prostate without damaging them is only about 30-50%.

Even with the nerve-sparing operation, nearly all men are impotent immediately following surgery. However, approximately 50% will regain some erectile function within a year of surgery (*Figure 6a*).

Younger patients more often remain potent after undergoing a nerve-sparing prostatectomy than older patients. In the most favorable reports, men between 50 and 60 have approximately a 75% chance of remaining potent, while men between the ages of 70 and 80 have only a 25% chance of remaining potent (*Figure 6b*).

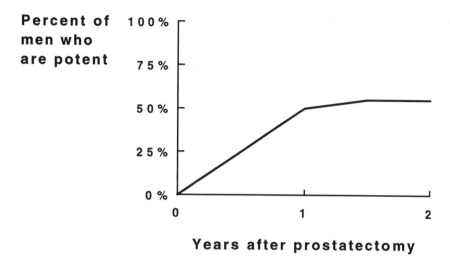

Figure 6a . The recovery of potency following prostatectomy.

The likelihood that a patient will maintain his potency varies according to different surgeons, reflecting both the skill of the surgeon and how doctors rate their success. Dr. Walsh reports that approximately 50% of his patients remain potent after the nerve-sparing prostatectomy. In contrast, a recent survey of Medicare patients treated throughout the United States found that only 10% of patients could still have erections.

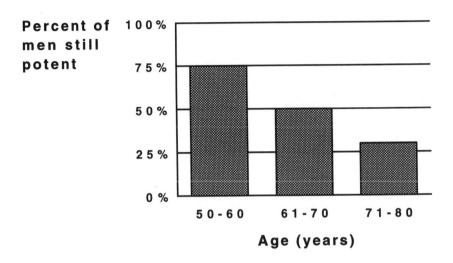

Figure 6b. Likelihood of preservation of sexual potency versus a patient's age at the time of prostatectomy.

Variation in the reported potency rates also reflects differences in how potency is defined by researchers. If a patient has only slightly less firm erections, most doctors would report that he is still potent. However, many patients have substantially less firm erections, that may or may not be sufficient for sexual intercourse. Researchers differ substantially when classifying such patients.

The likelihood of cure with surgery

PSA SHOULD GO DOWN TO ZERO

If a man's entire cancer is removed at the time of his surgery, his PSA reading should go down to zero. If any PSA is detectable, cancer probably remains. Cancer left behind is often not recognized at the time of surgery because the amount left is usually too small to be seen with the naked eye. When the prostate is examined under a microscope, doctors can often determine whether any cancer extended through the prostate capsule.

Sometimes a man's PSA is zero after surgery but rises several years later. In such cases, the amount of cancer left behind was so tiny that the PSA it produced was too small to detect. However, as the remaining cancer grows, it produces detectable PSA. The time required for minute amounts of cancer to grow large enough to produce detectable PSA explains why some men with residual cancer are not identified until several years after their operation.

The likelihood that a person can be surgically cured of cancer varies according to the stage of his cancer. The staging system is designed to identify which patients will have cancer limited to their prostate. Men with Stage A or B cancer are most likely to have cancer truly limited to the prostate, and are most likely to be cured by a prostatectomy. However, patients with Stage A or B cancers can be mis-staged. The cancer can be more extensive than appreciated based on the initial work-up tests. Even a small amount of cancer extending through the capsule will usually be left behind after surgery because it is impossible to remove a sizable margin of tissue around the prostate. The prostate is immediately adjacent to the rectum, bladder and pelvic bones. These structures cannot be removed along with the prostate to give a wider margin.

RESULTS NOT AS GOOD AS PREVIOUSLY BELIEVED

Long term PSA data following prostatectomy is still limited. The first study to include PSA information while analyzing cure rates was from the University of California, Los Angeles (UCLA). Within 5 years of surgery, approximately 30% of patients had evidence of cancer recurrence, based on detectable PSA. The cancers continued to recur after 5 years, with 60% of men having evidence of cancer recurrence 10 years after the operation (*Figure 6c*).

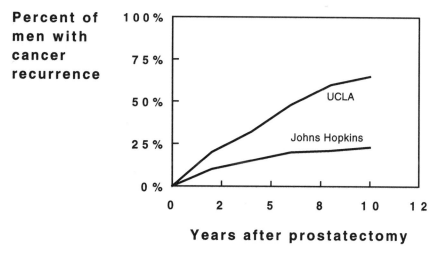

Figure 6c. The likelihood of cancer recurrence after prostatectomy for Stage A or B cancer.

With 10 year follow-up, only 40% of patients were still in remission. Moreover, after 10 years, some additional men may experience recurrence of their cancer. The actual cure rate in this group of patients is still not known.

The UCLA reports revealed higher failure rates than previously believed. Researchers at other major surgical centers have reported on the percent of men who appear cured by surgery. Probably the most carefully treated and most carefully analyzed group of surgery patients is from Dr. Patrick Walsh at Johns Hopkins University. Dr. Walsh has been very careful to select those patients most likely to have cancer that has not yet grown outside of the prostatic capsule. He does so based on digital rectal exams, PSA levels, and Gleason score, factors that help determine stage. In general, patients operated on by Dr. Walsh have a much lower PSA before their operations than any other group of men reported. In fact, approximately 40% of the men operated on by Dr. Walsh have normal PSAs. By limiting his patients to those with the lowest PSAs and lowest Gleason scores, his cure rates will be better than those achieved by less selective surgeons. Within 5 years of surgery, approximately 15% of the men operated on by Dr. Walsh have evidence of cancer recurrence, shown by a rising PSA. Ten years after surgery, approximately 20% of the men have evidence of cancer recurrence (*Figure 6c*). Therefore, the cure rate, looking at 10 years of follow-up after surgery, appears to be approximately 80%. Even after 10 years, however, a few more men will probably develop recurrence. The ultimate cure rate for this group of patients is still unknown.

EFFECT OF PSA AND GLEASON SCORE ON CHANCE FOR CURE

The PSA and Gleason score determine, to a large extent, the likelihood of cure from prostate cancer. A high PSA or Gleason score reveals a greater chance that some cancer has grown through the prostate capsule. That portion of protruding cancer will usually not be removed during surgery because very little tissue around the prostate is removed along with the prostate. Accordingly, men with a high Gleason score or PSA reading have less chance of being cured. The probability of cancer reappearing in men with a Gleason score of 8 or more is over 50% (*Figure 6d*).

Prostate cancer is more likely to reappear in those men who have a high PSA at the time of diagnosis. Men with a PSA greater than 20 have a 50% probability of having their cancer recur (*Figure 6e*).

Because of the higher cancer recurrence rate after surgery in patients with PSA above 20 or Gleason above 7, some doctors are reluctant to recommend surgery for this group of men. Unfortunately, the cure rates for such men do not appear any higher following radiation. The best treatment for these patients is still an issue of debate.

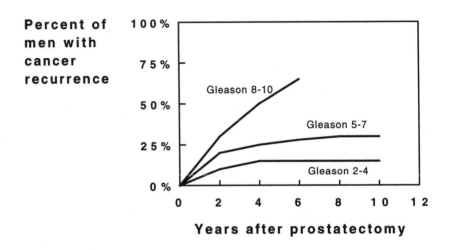

Figure 6d. The likelihood of cancer recurrence after prostatectomy for Stage A or B cancer, based on Gleason score of the tumor.

Radical prostatectomy compared to "watchful waiting"

Only one scientific trial has been performed to test the effectiveness of prostatectomy. Conducted at the Veteran's Administration hospitals, 95 patients with Stage A or B cancer were assigned to either surgery or no treatment. The study showed that men who had a prostatectomy had the same chance of being alive 15

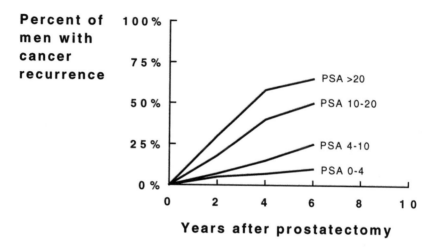

Figure 6e . The likelihood of cancer recurrence for Stage A or B cancer, based on pre-surgical PSA.

years after surgery as those who were not treated. However, the trial has been criticized for several reasons. Most importantly, the number of patients enrolled in the trial was too small to reliably show a statistical difference with prostatectomy. Such criticisms are valid. Two large trials are now being undertaken to test the long term cure rates of patients undergoing prostatectomy versus those given no treatment. One trial is to be run in the United States, and the other in Europe. Unfortunately, meaningful results from these trials will not be available until at least 2005.

Use of hormonal therapy to shrink cancer before surgery

Hormonal treatment shrinks a man's prostate by approximately 50% (see Chapter 10). Some surgeons advocate the use of hormonal ablation for several months prior to a prostatectomy, in the hope of making removal of the prostate easier. While there is some rationale for this use of hormonal treatment, there is still no clear evidence that it will increase the likelihood of being cured. Many physicians do not currently recommend this additional therapy, but it is a valid option.

If surgery does not remove all of the cancer

In patients who develop measurable PSA after surgery, some cancer may have been left at the margins of their prostates. Alternatively, minute amounts of cancer may have spread to other areas of the body, even though it is not detectable by bone scan or by lymph node removal during the operation.

If PSA is detectable and rising after the patient's prostatectomy, a bone scan is routinely done to make sure no metastatic disease exists. If the bone scan is negative, it is possible that the cancer remains only in the prostatic region. In these situations, further surgery would not be advisable. Options to consider at this point are hormone therapy, radiation or simply watchful waiting. A second attempt at a cure is called "salvage" treatment, because it is an attempt to salvage a cure after an initial failure.

SALVAGE TREATMENTS FOR FAILED SURGERY

If men with rising PSAs after prostatectomy begin hormone therapy, the residual cancer will shrink down, making the PSA undetectable. Some physicians advocate using hormonal therapy as soon as PSA is detectable after prostatectomy, believing that it will cure some patients, or at least "slow the cancer down." However, this rationale is questionable. Although hormonal therapy will cause the PSA to decrease, the effect is usually temporary. No firm evidence exists to show that hormone therapy can cure men with recurrent prostate cancer.

A second option for men with detectable PSA after prostatectomy is to receive radiation at the prostatic region, in the hope of destroying any cancer that might remain there. Radiation administered after surgery is similar to the treatment that is given to patients as their primary treatment, but the dose is decreased by approximately 20%. The PSA usually decreases, but not always back to zero, where it should be if the radiation destroys all remaining cancer. Approximately 30% of men with detectable PSA post-prostatectomy appear to still be curable with radiation, evidenced by the fact that their PSAs go back to zero and stay there. Some patients cannot be cured because some cancers are resistant to radiation or will have metastasized.

While the use of radiation in men who have cancer recurrence after prostatectomy appears to offer a second chance at a cure, there may be some increased chance of urinary incontinence. Fortunately, the risk appears to be small. For men with full urinary control after their surgery, radiation rarely causes the loss of that control. However, for men who have not regained full urinary control, radiation could retard a return to full control. For this reason, some doctors suggest delaying any radiation for 6 months or so after a prostatectomy. In addition, the radiation may adversely affect a man's ability to retain his sexual potency after surgery.

7

External radiation

External radiation has been widely used to treat prostate cancer for nearly 40 years. There have been a series of technical improvements during that time.

What is radiation

Radiation (x-rays) is a form of energy similar to visible light. X-rays are composed of such high energy that they penetrate tissue. As x-rays pass through the body they are gradually absorbed.

Radiation can be generated from radioactive metals (cobalt) or produced electrically from a machine called a linear accelerator. X-rays from a linear accelerator are higher energy and can be directed more accurately than those from a cobalt machine. The use of a linear accelerator is preferable for prostate cancer treatment.

How radiation works

In the center of each cell is the nucleus. Inside the nucleus is the DNA. This DNA stores information a cell needs to carry on its usual functions. That information is continually used to direct the production of proteins that a cell needs.

If radiation is directed at the body, some of the radiation is absorbed by cells and damages the DNA. Radiation damage to DNA kills cells. In general, cancer cells are more sensitive to radiation than are normal cells so the radiation dose needed to destroy cancer is unlikely to cause serious damage to surrounding, normal tissues. However, the difference in radiation sensitivity is small and therefore, the radiation dose needed to destroy prostate cancer carries some possibility of damaging the adjacent rectum or bladder.

How external radiation is given

PLANNING

Delivery of good quality radiation treatments is a sophisticated procedure. Because each man's prostate and surrounding organs are unique in size and shape, the radiation beams must be designed specifically for each patient. To do so, the patient goes to the radiation facility several days before his treatments begin for a planning session.

To make the patient's position on the treatment machine reproducible for the daily treatments, marks are made on his skin at the front, back and sides of his pelvis. The marks are made permanent by the placement of several, pinhead size tattoos on the patient's skin. These skin marks are used to align the patient each day to a set of laser beams mounted in the treatment room. A custom-made plastic mold can also be used to help keep the patient in the same position each day. Once the patient is properly positioned, a CT scan is performed.

From the CT scan, the position of the patient's prostate, seminal vesicles, rectum and bladder are outlined. This information determines how the radiation beams should enter the body, as well as the shape of the beams. The radiation is given from several different directions. The beams intersect and form a high-dose region around the prostate. This focuses the radiation on the prostate without over-radiating adjacent portions of the bladder and rectum.

The process of designing the radiation beam configuration is called "simulation" because it simulates the actual treatments. The design of the beams is arrived at jointly by the radiation oncologist in collaboration with a medical physicist.

THE TREATMENT ITSELF

The patient is placed in the same position each day, either face up or face down (*Figure 7a*). A radiation treatment takes approximately 10 minutes. The treatment is administered by a radiation technologist, who has had 2-4 years of specialized schooling in radiation therapy.

For the daily treatment the patient should expect to be in the radiation facility for an hour, allowing time to get undressed, to be properly positioned, to receive

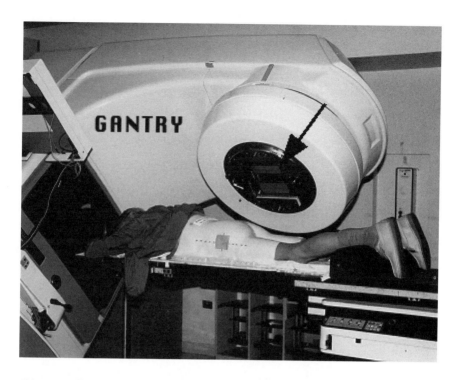

Figure 7a. A patient on the treatment table of a linear accelerator. The plastic mold helps keep him in the proper position. The main portion of the machine (gantry) can rotate around to direct the radiation beam from different angles. The radiation beam itself exits from the collimator (large arrow).

the treatment and to get dressed. The radiation treatment itself is completely painless—it cannot be felt.

Radiation is given in small daily doses

Radiation is given in small daily doses, five days per week. Splitting the radiation into small daily doses decreases the chance of injury to adjacent, normal tissues.

Once a course of treatment is started, the patient should finish the course with minimal interruption. During a seven to eight week course, often one or more treatments is missed. Reasons commonly include machine maintenance for a day, or bad weather. If a treatment is missed, it is made up at the end of the treatment course. Delaying treatment up to five days has no discernible effect on the chance of being cured. However, interruptions of more than five treatments during the radiation course should be avoided.

How much radiation is given

Radiation is measured in a unit called the Gray (Gy), an amount of radiation analogous to a Watt of light. (The old unit of measure was the "rad"; 1 Gray = 100 rads.) The typical daily dose of radiation is 1.8 to 2.0 Gy (or 180 to 200 rads).

The radiation dose given, in large part, determines the likelihood of destroying a cancer. Higher doses of radiation have a higher likelihood of destroying a cancer. Unfortunately, there are limits to the amount of radiation that can be given safely, as too much radiation to the adjacent portions of the rectum or bladder can lead to complications. Until the mid 1980's, it was believed that the maximum dose that could be safely given to the prostate was 70 Gray. A maximum dose of 70 Gray was established from studies in the 1970s. With the technology available at that time, doses of more than 70 Gray were associated with a higher risk of serious complications. However, those studies were done without current, improved technology, including high quality CT scans, MRI scans and computer-aided radiation planning.

CONFORMAL THERAPY

Since the 1970s, substantial improvements in the accuracy of radiation delivery have been made. Previously, prostate position and shape were estimated from simple, two dimensional x-rays. In the 1980s computer-aided methodology was devised to facilitate the design of more accurate, tailored radiation treatments. Part of this technical evolution has been the use of CT scan images to define a man's prostate in three dimensions, and then to conform the radiation to the shape of his prostate. Use of sophisticated computer-assisted planning procedures to shape the radiation dose more accurately are referred to as "3-D" or "conformal" radiation. These techniques are a significant technical advance in radiation therapy.

HIGHER DOSES APPEAR SAFER

Because of technological improvements and a better understanding of how prostate cancer grows, researchers at many medical centers have been routinely treating patients to doses higher than 70 Gray. As of 1994, there appears to be little or no increased risk of complications with higher doses, up to 80 Gy.

THERE IS NO POINT IN TREATING THE ENTIRE PELVIS

It has been shown that for Stage A or B cancer patients, highly focused radiation is usually more appropriate than radiating a large part of the pelvis. Until the mid-1980s, it was common practice to treat a very generous area around the patient's prostate. This was done in the hope that any cancer which might have spread to the lymph nodes could still be eradicated. But, in the '80s, a large, experimental trial run in the United States showed that treatment to wide areas beyond the patient's prostate was no better than focusing the radiation only on the prostate. Consequently, radiation is now usually focused on the prostate and seminal vesicles, with only an inch or so of margin. By limiting the area that receives a high radiation dose the total dose to the patient's prostate can be increased.

LEGAL FEARS

The use of higher radiation doses, using more sophisticated treatment methods appears to be safe. Almost certainly more can be gained than lost by increasing the dose to 75 Gy or higher. Nevertheless, some radiation doctors are reluctant to exceed standard radiation doses for fear of legal action should a complication occur. This is probably an area where fear of legal repercussions could substantially decrease a treatment's curative potential. If the low cure rates achieved with conventional radiation doses are to be increased, both doctors and patients must be willing to raise the radiation dose. Most large radiation facilities already have more advanced technology to do some form of 3D treatment. As more experience is gained with the better technology, higher doses will probably become standard.

Neutrons and protons

As described previously, conventional radiation (x-rays) is a form of energy similar to visible light. The energy is in the form of tiny packets called "photons." Alternative forms of radiation have been developed, in the hope that they might be more effective than photons. Neutrons and protons are types of radiation that are composed of tiny particles, rather than being pure energy packets.

Neutrons have a theoretical advantage over photons, in that they are more effective against portions of cancer that have a lower oxygen content than normal. Neutrons have been studied in scientific trials, and have shown substantially higher cancer control rates for advanced tumors. There has been a higher likelihood of intestinal complications compared to treatment with conventional radiation, but that is probably related to technical problems that can be solved. Many radiation oncologists are skeptical that the results are truly better, but further studies are warranted.

Protons have a theoretical advantage over photons, in that they can be focused somewhat better. Scientific trials to date, however, have not shown a clear advantage for protons over photons. Like neutrons, further studies are warranted.

Who is eligible for external radiation

Because radiation does not involve anesthesia or the risk of an operation, nearly all men can safely tolerate the treatment. The chance of being cured by this treatment is highest for small cancers (Stages A or B). More advanced cancers (Stage C) are usually treated with radiation, although the chance for cure is less.

Men whose cancer has metastasized to the bones or the lymph nodes cannot be cured with radiation. They should have radiation to the prostate only if the cancer within the prostate is causing problems by obstructing the urine passage, pushing into the rectum, or causing discomfort in the rectum. Radiation is commonly used to treat cancer that has metastasized to bone, to relieve associated bone pain.

Usual side effects of external radiation

A radiation course lasts seven to nine weeks, depending on the total dose given. During the first two weeks, most men will not experience any side effects. After about two weeks of treatment, the cumulative dose of radiation begins to cause inflammation of the prostate and the part of the rectum immediately behind the patient's prostate. This inflammation can cause radiation-related symptoms of irritation and more frequent bowel movements.

GENERAL SIDE EFFECTS

Side effects, which can occur with radiation treatment to other parts of the body, are unusual with prostate radiation. Some patients may experience fatigue. This is probably related to the tension of going through the daily treatments, rather than the radiation itself. Patients should not experience hair loss, nausea or vomiting.

IN PERSPECTIVE

A man working full-time prior to treatment would probably not miss work due to radiation side effects.

Usually the only substantial effect on one's lifestyle is the time required for the daily trips to the facility.

URINE SYMPTOMS

After two weeks of treatment, patients usually experience more frequent urination. Frequent urination is most noticeable during the night when one wakes up and has to get out of bed to urinate. Patients also commonly notice a mild burning sensation upon urination. Urinary symptoms usually plateau about three weeks after starting radiation, and usually do not get progressively worse as the treatments continue. Urinary symptoms generally subside a couple of weeks after finishing radiation.

RECTAL SYMPTOMS

Rectal irritation is common among radiation patients. It can start within two or three weeks of starting treatment, and lasts two to three weeks after treatment finishes. Rectal irritation results from radiation to the part of the rectum immediately adjacent to the back of the prostate, as that area will receive almost as much radiation as the prostate.

In addition to a feeling of rectal irritation, patients commonly have more frequent bowel movements, perhaps two to three per day, rather than one a day.

In the past, when radiation was given to the entire pelvis, patients often developed diarrhea during treatment. Now radiation treatment is usually focused on the prostate and diarrhea is unusual.

Complications of external radiation

While the usual side effects of external radiation are mild and quickly reversible, some chance of more serious, permanent complications exists. Potential long term complications of radiation include urinary incontinence, rectal damage and sexual impotence. These serious complications usually occur from six to 24 months after completing the radiation treatments. The delay is due to the time required to develop radiation-related weakening of the tissues.

URINE INCONTINENCE

Urinary incontinence refers to any difficulty holding one's urine, from dribbling a few drops with heavy lifting, to total loss of control. The chance of any degree of incontinence after radiation is low. So low, in fact, a precise estimate of the risk is difficult. The likelihood is approximately 1 in 100 patients. This risk may be higher in patients who have undergone prior prostate surgery (TURP).

RECTAL DAMAGE

Radiation damage to the rectum is the most serious, but uncommon, complication of radiation. Because the prostate is located immediately adjacent to the rectum, separated only by one eighth of an inch, that part of the rectum will receive as much radiation as the prostate. Fortunately, the portion of the rectum adjacent to the prostate only comprises a small portion of the entire rectum.

High-dose radiation to a small area of the rectum is generally safe. However, there is a small possibility that the rectum of some patients will not tolerate the radiation and these patients may develop inflammation which can lead to rectal bleeding. This bleeding is painless and usually occurs when having bowel movements. It is due to the pressure from stool passing through the rectum. Such bleeding will usually stop spontaneously within one to three years. Medication may help this condition to heal faster than it would spontaneously. The percentage of men who experience rectal bleeding after radiation is about 5 in 100. The likelihood could be higher with very high dose, conformal radiation.

Rarely, in severe cases of rectal bleeding, a colostomy may be necessary, whereby the patient's lower intestines are diverted to a bag worn on the skin. This is necessary in cases where there is excessive bleeding, or when a hole develops between the rectum and the urine passage (urethra). If a colostomy is needed, the radiation damage may gradually heal, so that in some men, the colostomy can be reversed. Such healing might take several years.

The chance of having a severe rectal complication after radiation is less than 1%. In fact, it is so uncommon that it is impossible to give a more exact number.

SEXUAL IMPOTENCE

The most common radiation related complication is sexual impotence. Impotence refers to the inability to have an erection, while the desire for sex is unchanged. Radiation-related impotence is a result of damage to the small blood vessels and the nerves responsible for erections. Unfortunately, impotence due to radiation is usually permanent. Also common after radiation is a decrease in the volume of a patient's ejaculate fluid.

The likelihood of developing impotence following external radiation rises over time, reflecting a combination of late radiation changes and the natural effects of aging. One year after radiation, only about 10% of men become impotent. However, after 5 years approximately 50% of men will develop impotence (*Figure 7b*). Men should remember that there are several effective methods to restore useful erections (see Chapter 12).

SPERM COULD BE DAMAGED

When treating prostate cancer, radiation is not aimed directly at the testicles. However, a small amount of scatter radiation reaches the testicles. The testicles still produce male hormone (testosterone) normally, but some damage to the sperm from the scatter radiation is possible. Most men who develop prostate cancer are beyond the age of wanting to father children. Those men who are considering fathering more children should bank sperm before undergoing radiation treatments.

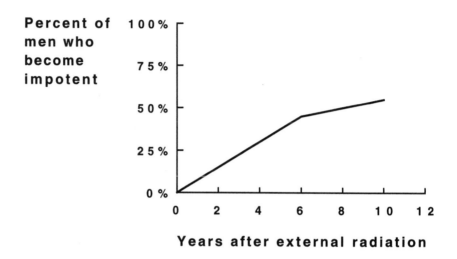

Figure 7b. Percent of men who become impotent follow-ing external radiation.

The likelihood of cure

As discussed in Chapter 5, the likelihood of cure by external radiation is substantially less than what was assumed before the introduction of PSA. The PSA test detects cancer recurrence much sooner than was previously possible.

As with other methods of treatment, the likelihood of being cured by external radiation is heavily influenced by the cancer stage, Gleason score, and PSA. Of all patients with Stage A or B cancer, approximately 50% are cured with external radiation. Men with larger, Stage C cancer are less likely to be cured (*Figure 7c*).

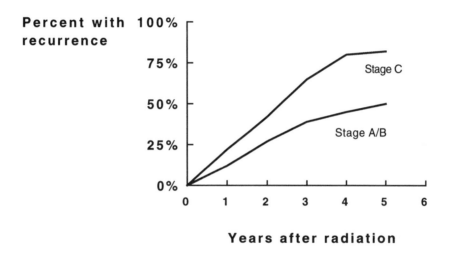

Figure 7c. Cancer recurrence after external radiation for Stage A, B or C cancer.

The PSA level at the time of diagnosis is the best indicator of the likelihood a man will be cured of prostate cancer. A higher PSA usually indicates a more advanced cancer and, therefore, one less likely to be eradicated by radiation. The cancer recurrence rate increases with increasing PSA at the time of diagnosis. Men who have a PSA in the normal range are most likely to be cured. The recurrence rate is higher in men with a PSA between four and ten, and goes up progressively as the PSA rises (*Figure 7d*).

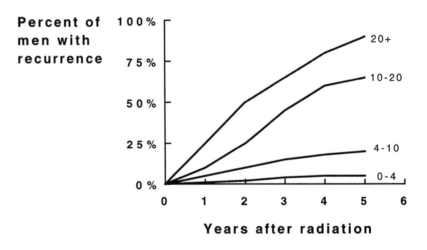

Figure 7d. Percent of men with cancer recurrence after radiation for Stage A or B cancer, based on their pretreatment PSA of 0-4, 4-10, 10-20 or greater than 20.

The Gleason score is another predictor of the probability a patient can be cured by radiation. Men whose

Gleason scores are lower are more likely to be cured (*Figure 7e*).

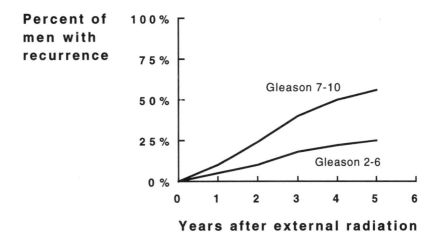

Figure 7e. Cancer recurrence after external radiation for Stages A or B, with Gleason of 2-6 or Gleason 7-10.

Use of hormonal therapy to shrink cancer before radiation

Three months of hormonal treatment will shrink a patient's prostate to about half its original size (see Chapter 11). It has been argued that combining the shrinking effect of hormonal therapy with the effect of radiation might offer a better chance of destroying a patient's cancer, than using either method alone. Several studies have suggested some benefit to using hormonal therapy in addition to external radiation. Hormonal therapy, combined with radiation, delays recurrence. However, men who received hormonal therapy did not necessarily live longer.

When hormonal treatment is used along with radiation, it appears that the treatment keeps any remaining cancer in remission, but may not eradicate the remaining cancer. In effect, then, hormonal ablation may not actually increase the chance of being cured. The issue is still being studied.

One reason to use hormone ablation treatment before external radiation is that shrinking the prostate makes it easier to include the entire prostate in the high radiation dose region. By making the prostate smaller, less surrounding tissues are included in the high dose radiation area, presumably resulting in less chance of complications. But, use of hormone ablation to reduce the chance of complications probably makes sense only for men with a very enlarged prostate.

If radiation does not destroy all of the cancer

If a patient's cancer is destroyed by external radiation, his PSA should gradually fall to very low levels, usually within 12 months. If his PSA falls to less than 1.0, it is very likely that the cancer is completely, permanently eradicated. If his PSA is above 2 at 12 months after radiation, some cancer likely remains. If a man's prostate cancer is not eradicated, the first sign is that his PSA begins to rise again at some time after treatment.

If his PSA begins to rise after treatment, a bone scan should be done to determine if metastatic disease is present. If the bone scan shows no metastatic cancer, the residual cancer may be confined to the prostate. In general, if a man's PSA rises very slowly after radiation (over one to three years), any residual cancer is probably still contained within his prostate. Deciding what to do in such situations is difficult. Ideally, one would try a second time to be cured, either with surgery or radiation. A second attempt at cure is called "salvage" treatment because it is an attempt to salvage a cure after an initial failure to do so.

SALVAGE TREATMENTS FOR FAILED EXTERNAL RADIATION

Re-treatment with external radiation is not practical. It carries a very high risk of complications, and is very unlikely to work, since the first course of radiation did not.

Considerable interest has been shown in using implant radiation as a salvage treatment in men who have failed external radiation treatment. Implants can give a high dose of radiation, with relatively little additional radiation to the rectum. While there is some appeal to this idea, the risk of serious complications probably outweighs the potential benefits of salvage treatment. As of 1996, very little has been reported in the medical literature about this alternative. And what has been reported does not sound encouraging. If one decides to have salvage treatment, prostatectomy would probably be preferable to implantation.

Several research reports have been compiled on the use of salvage prostatectomy for men not cured by external radiation. The operation is the same as that done if a person had never had radiation, but is technically more difficult. The likelihood of complications, including urinary incontinence and impotence, is substantially higher. Urine incontinence, in particular, occurs in about 50% of patients who have had radiation prior to prostatectomy, and the incidence of sexual impotence is probably close to 100%. Most worrisome about the use of salvage prostatectomy, however, is that only about 10-20% of such patients appear to be cured. Most doctors are not enthusiastic in recommending salvage prostatectomy, because the chance for cure is low, and the chance for complications is high. For a man who is otherwise in good health, the potential benefit may outweigh the risk.

Cryosurgery, another treatment method, uses freezing probes inserted into the prostate to freeze cancerous tissue. It is being used for treating men whose cancer has returned after radiation. There is very little data to date regarding its effectiveness or possible complications.

8

Implant radiation

Implant radiation refers to direct placement of radioactive pellets into the prostate. "Brachytherapy" is a Greek word for implant radiation. The pellets are inserted through hollow needles, precisely into the prostate. Radioactive implants deliver a highly concentrated radiation dose to the prostate, with a relatively low dose to the adjacent normal organs.

The idea is not new

The concept of using radioactive implants is not new. They were performed with old-fashioned radium needles in 1917, at what is now Memorial Sloan-Kettering Cancer Center in New York City. Despite their early theoretical appeal, until recently the technology did not exist to perform implants accurately. In the 1980s, the adaptation of ultrasound and computerized tomography (CT scans) for implants led to a resurgence in their use. Ultrasound and CT scanning allow precise planning of where the needles should go, and can be used to monitor insertion to insure the needles are placed properly before actually placing the pellets.

Planning the implant

To plan an implant, images of the patient's prostate are taken several days prior to the implant using ultrasound or CT. Those images are entered into a computer and used to determine how many pellets will be needed and where each pellet should be placed.

Performing the implant

General or spinal anesthesia can be used. Once anesthesia is started the patient is placed on his back, on an operating table. A needle guide template is mounted against the skin between the legs and hollow needles are inserted through the guiding template into the prostate (*Figure 8a*). The patch of skin between the legs and behind the scrotum is called the perineum, so that prostate implants done with needles inserted through that skin are called "transperineal implants."

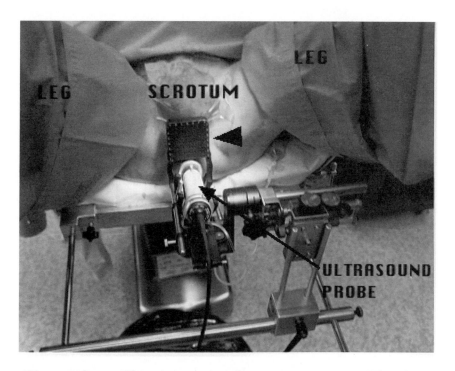

Figure 8a. This is an implant procedure. The large arrowhead points to the template through which the needles are inserted into the prostate. Radioactive seeds are then inserted through the hollow needles. (Courtesy of Peter Grimm, D.O.)

During the procedure, the needle positions are checked with x-rays and/or ultrasound to determine if they are in the right place. If they are not, the needles are removed, the guide template is repositioned, and the needles are re-inserted. Once the needles are properly positioned, the pellets are injected through the needles as the needles are withdrawn. This results in an array of radioactive seeds distributed throughout the prostate (*Figure 8b*).

The entire implant procedure takes about 60 minutes. It is usually done as an outpatient procedure, meaning that the patient comes into the hospital in the morning, has the procedure, and is sent home several hours later. A catheter (a thin flexible tube) is inserted through the penis and into the bladder during the implant, but is taken out before the patient goes home.

Some urinary burning occurs for at least one or two days afterwards, but patients rarely require pain medicines. During the first night after the implant, patients usually have frequent urination (every hour or so), due to irritation caused by the needle insertion. Men commonly pass some blood in their urine and ejaculation fluid for several days afterwards. Excessive bleeding almost never occurs. Antibiotics are usually prescribed, but may not be necessary.

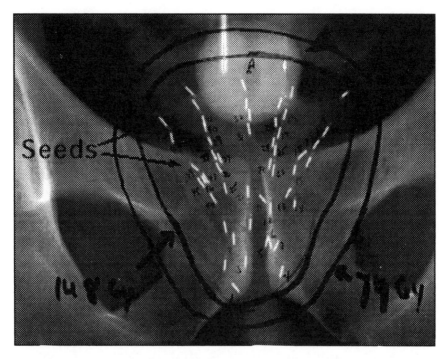

Figure 8b. An x-ray taken after an implant, showing the seeds distributed throughout the region of the prostate. The large arrowhead points to a balloon (filled with dye) attached to the end of a catheter, inserted through the penis into the bladder. The curved lines show the calculated radiation doses around the seed array.

Men are cautioned to avoid heavy lifting for several days afterwards. However, most are able to return to work within two days following the implant.

Permanent implants

Radioactive pellets can be inserted either temporarily or permanently. Permanent implants give off radiation over several months, until no more radiation is left. The metal casings are never removed. They are not reactive with body tissues and there is no known adverse effect from their being left in place. These casings are not large enough to be detected by metal detectors at airports and do not interfere with MRI scans.

Permanent implants are more commonly used than temporary ones. The primary advantage of permanent implants is that patients can go home several hours after implantation, rather than staying several nights in the hospital, as is the case for temporary implants.

Iodine or palladium for permanent implants

Two types of radioactive pellets are used for permanent implants. Both have shown promising results. Radioactive iodine (I-125) has been used for treatment of many cancer types since the 1950s. Radioactive palladium (Pd-103) is a newer type of pellet. Palladium has a shorter half-life than iodine, meaning that the radiation dose is given off faster (12 months with iodine versus 3 months for palladium). It has been argued that because the radiation dose is delivered more rapidly, palladium might be more effective against rapidly-growing cancers (those cancers with a higher Gleason score) . Conversely, mathematical studies suggest that the lower radiation dose rate of iodine is better for slower growing cancers (those with a lower Gleason score). This issue is still being studied.

Temporary Implants

For temporary implants, hollow plastic tubes (catheters) are inserted through the skin between the patient's legs into the prostate. Radioactive pellets are then inserted inside the tubes and left in place for several days. Afterwards, the pellets and hollow tubes are removed. These implants are done with pellets of radioactive iridium (Ir-192).

Temporary placement of radioactive seeds is probably equally effective as permanent implants. However, temporary implants require a three to five day hospital stay. Also, patients must remain relatively still in bed so that the tubes holding the iridium in place do not move. Because of the practical constraints of temporary implants, they are less commonly used.

Combining implants with external radiation

The high dose of implant radiation is limited to the prostate itself and a small rim of tissue around the prostate. Accordingly, implants are used primarily for Stage A or small Stage B cancers. Stage C cancers, by definition, have already grown through the prostate capsule and this protrusion may not be covered by radiation from an implant.

Because Stage C cancers extend beyond the prostate, they are generally treated with external radiation. However, interest is growing in treating Stage C or large Stage B cancers with a combination of implant plus external radiation. The rationale is that the implant will give a high, concentrated radiation dose to the cancer within the prostate, while the external radiation will cover any smaller areas of cancer that have protruded outside of the prostate.

The idea of combining external radiation with implantation is conceptually appealing, especially because the cure rates with external radiation alone for larger Stage B cancers and Stage C cancers are not high.

Early results from centers using a combination of implant plus external radiation look very promising. However, it is not clear if the combination will prove better than high dose, conformal 3D external radiation alone.

Which patients are appropriate

GENERAL HEALTH CONSIDERATIONS

Most patients can physically tolerate the implantation procedure. Only light anesthesia is needed. Men with a history of heart disease or stroke should have a thorough medical evaluation before proceeding with implantation. An evaluation might include a cardiac stress test.

Men who have had the central portion of their prostate removed (TURP) in the past, may be at increased risk of urine incontinence after implantation. A CT scan or MRI scan often determine how much tissue had been removed with a previous TURP. If only a small amount of tissue was removed, it is probably safe to have an implant.

Men with a very enlarged prostate or those who have substantial difficulty passing their urine before treatment may have more severe urinary symptoms following implantation. Some doctors have prescribed two months of hormone treatment prior to the implant to shrink the prostate. The benefit of hormone treatment prior to implantation is not clearly proven.

WHAT STAGES ARE APPROPRIATE

Implantation alone is used for Stage A or small Stage B tumors, those usually confined to the prostate. Men with more advanced cancers are unlikely to be cured with implant alone because the implant does not radiate enough area around the prostate to destroy cancer that may have grown outside the prostate capsule.

Men with larger Stage B cancers, a high Gleason score or a high PSA are more likely to have cancer that extends outside of the capsule. Men with a Gleason score of 8 or more, or a PSA above 10, should generally be treated with high dose external radiation, or a combination of implant plus external radiation.

Stage C cancers by definition extend beyond the prostate. These patients should be treated with high dose external radiation or a combination of implant plus external radiation.

Usual side effects of implantation

GENERAL SIDE EFFECTS

General radiation side effects are unusual with prostate implants, because the radiation is limited to such a small area of the body. Fatigue can occur, but is usually minimal. No hair loss, nausea, vomiting or diarrhea should occur.

URINARY SYMPTOMS

The urinary side effects of implantation are similar to those of external radiation, but are more intense. Implant radiation induces inflammation of the prostate and that portion of the urine passage (urethra) that passes through the prostate. Inflammation of the patient's prostate and urethra leads to frequent urination and sometimes a burning sensation upon urination. Frequent urination is most intense at night, when men commonly will have to urinate every one to two hours for several months after the implant.

Also, men commonly have more urgency to urinate, so that when the need is felt, one has to do so quickly. These urinary symptoms are usually limited to the first several months after implantation, when the radiation dose is at its highest.

With iodine, urinary symptoms peak at about four to six weeks after the implant, and gradually subside over the next 3 to 12 months. With palladium, patients' symptoms may start sooner and resolve sooner.

RECTAL SYMPTOMS

Implant radiation causes inflammation of a one-inch patch of the patient's rectum, adjacent to the prostate. A feeling of rectal irritation when having a bowel movement is common, lasting for several months after the implant. More frequent bowel movements (two to three per day) are common. Rectal irritation starts within two or three weeks of the implant, and lasts three to six months. Diarrhea should not occur.

PUTTING IT IN PERSPECTIVE

Men working full-time prior to the implant are unlikely to miss work because of the radiation side effects, which are usually not substantial enough to keep patients from their normal activities. However, radiation symptoms following implantation are usually more marked than with external radiation because more radiation is delivered with the implant.

Complications of implantation

While the usual side effects of implant radiation are mild and reversible, there is some chance of more serious, permanent complications. Potential long term complications include urinary incontinence, rectal damage and sexual impotence. These serious complications usually occur from six to 24 months after the implant.

URINE INCONTINENCE

Urinary incontinence refers to any difficulty holding one's urine, from dribbling of a few drops with physical exertion, to total loss of control. In men without prior prostate surgery, the likelihood of incontinence after implantation is probably less than 1%. Incontinence is usually limited to patients who have had a TURP (surgical removal of the central portion of their prostate) in the past.

RECTAL COMPLICATIONS

Implants deliver a high dose of radiation to the patient's rectum that is immediately against the back of the prostate. This spot of rectum develops a substantial radiation reaction, which may result in intermittent rectal bleeding. Such bleeding shows up as a spot of bright red blood on the toilet paper, especially after a hard bowel movement that irritates the rectal lining. This bleeding usually heals by itself in about one to two years. Minor rectal bleeding probably occurs in about 5% of men, and rarely requires medication.

Serious rectal complications requiring surgical intervention are rare. A small percentage of men have developed ulceration of the rectum overlying the prostate. Such ulcerations usually heal within one to two years. The necessity for surgical repair (colostomy) is rare. In experienced hands, the likelihood of a serious rectal complication is less than 1 in 100.

SEXUAL FUNCTION

The prostate is a sex organ. Its function is to provide fluid to help transport sperm. Therefore, high dose radiation of the prostate can affect sexual function.

Approximately one-third of men report a brief pain or burning sensation with ejaculation, occurring for three to six months after implantation. Men commonly notice they have less fluid with ejaculation. Patients still contemplating having children should bank sperm beforehand.

Implant radiation can cause sexual impotence. Impotence is the inability to have an erection, while the desire for sex is unchanged. Radiation induced impotence probably results from damage to the small nerves or blood vessels that normally induce erections. Impotence due to radiation is usually permanent.

Only approximately 5% of men develop impotence within one year after implantation. However, the likelihood of impotence increases as time passes, reflecting a combination of late radiation changes and natural aging in men. Five years after implantation, about three fourths of patients are still potent. The potency rates after implantation are higher than that after prostatectomy or external radiation (*Figure 8c*).

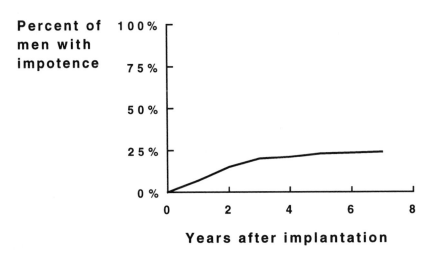

Percent of men with impotence

Figure 8c. Effect of implantation on potency. Approximately 20% of men who are potent before implant will develop impotence within 5 years after treatment.

The effect of implant radiation on potency is related to one's age at the time of implantation. Men under 60 at the time of implant are much more likely to keep their potency.

Effective remedies to restore erections for men who become impotent after implantation are available (see Chapter 11).

Likelihood of cure

Modern implant techniques were perfected in the 1980s. As of 1996, several investigators have accumulated 5 to 10 year results for men implanted for Stage A or B cancers. Results following implantation are similar to those following prostatectomy. Overall, approximately 60 to 90% of men are cancer-free, depending on the pre-treatment PSA and Gleason score (*Figure 8d*).

While the results are very encouraging, 5 to 7 years is still a short amount of time for a cancer that grows as slowly as prostate cancer. Another 5 to 10 years is needed to be confident that the cure rate is as high as it appears in 1995. In the meantime, it can be said that results with modern implants are similar to, or better than, surgery or external radiation, when the results of each treatment form are compared at similar times.

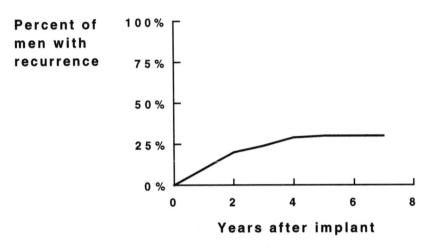

Figure 8d. Cancer recurrence in first 7 years after radioactive iodine implantation for Stage A or B cancer.

Effect of Gleason score and PSA on cure

The likelihood of cure by implantation is influenced by the extent of disease at diagnosis. Men with a higher Gleason score or PSA have a lower chance of being cured (*Figure 8e*).

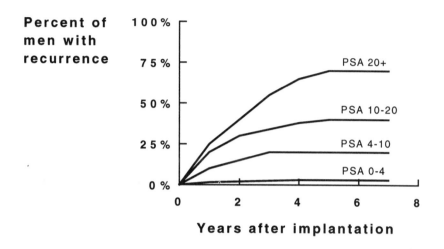

Figure 8e. Cancer recurrence after radioactive iodine implantation for Stage A or B cancer, based on the PSA level before treatment.

If implant radiation does not destroy all of the cancer

If cancer is destroyed by implantation, a patient's PSA should gradually fall to very low levels, usually within 12 months. If a cancer is not destroyed, the PSA falls, but then begins to rise again. If his PSA is above 2 at 12 months after having an implant, there is a high chance that some cancer remains.

If a man's PSA is found to be rising after an implant procedure, a bone scan should be done to determine if metastatic disease is present. If the scan shows no metastatic cancer, the cancer may still be confined to the prostate. In general, if a patient's PSA rises very slowly, the cancer is more likely confined to the prostate, and not yet spread outside of the prostate. Deciding what to do in these situations is difficult. Ideally, one would like to try a second treatment, either with prostatectomy or radiation.

SALVAGE TREATMENT FOR FAILED IMPLANTS

A salvage prostatectomy after seed implantation is the same as would be done if a person had never had radiation, but it is technically more difficult. The likelihood of complications, including urinary incontinence and impotence, is higher. Urine incontinence in particular, may occur in approximately 50% of patients. The likelihood of sexual impotence is probably close to 100%.

Little data has been reported on the use of prostatectomy for patients not cured by implantation. From what is known, probably only about 10 to 20% of such patients will be cured. The likelihood of cure with salvage prostatectomy is low because the same men who are not cured by an implant are probably the same ones who would not have been cured by a prostatectomy as their first treatment, i.e.: those whose cancer has grown beyond the prostate.

Most doctors have low enthusiasm for salvage prostatectomy, because the chance for cure is low, and the chance for complications is relatively high. For a man who is otherwise in good health the potential benefit might outweigh the risk.

For men not cured with implantation, re-treatment with external radiation is not practical. It would carry a high risk of rectal complications, and would probably not be curative.

Interest has been shown in using a second implant as a salvage treatment in men who have failed a first implant. While this idea has some appeal, it is unlikely the benefits of salvage treatment with re-implantation would outweigh the risk of serious complications. An exception to this scenario would be men who had a technically inadequate implant the first time, in which the seeds were not all in the prostate or the total number of pellets was too small. Even then, such men would face a substantial risk of complications from a second implant. If one were to have salvage treatment, prostatectomy is probably the preferable option.

Another consideration for salvage treatment is cryosurgery (Chapter 9). It is primarily being used to treat men whose cancer has recurred after radiation. There is little data regarding its effectiveness or the possible complications of this method. However, it is worth looking into as an option if implant radiation fails.

9

Cryotherapy

Cryotherapy (commonly called "cryo") is the use of freezing to kill cancer cells. The idea has been tried for a variety of cancer types in the past, with mixed results. Like brachytherapy, however, recent technical improvements have allowed more precise use of the technique.

How cryotherapy is done

To perform cryotherapy, 3-6 hollow needles are inserted into the prostate using ultrasound guidance, similar to an implant procedure. Once the needles are in their proper position, liquid nitrogen is run through the needles, freezing the tissue around the needles. The procedure is done with spinal or general anesthesia.

A catheter with warm water running through it is kept in the urethra during the procedure to protect the lining of the urine passage from freezing.

Freezing of the prostatic tissue can be seen as an advancing dark circle on the ultrasound screen, and the liquid nitrogen flow is stopped when the edge of the freezing zone reaches the periphery of the prostate.

The entire procedure takes about 2 hours to perform, and the patient usually stays in the hospital for one night. Patients generally go home with a suprapubic catheter (a urine drainage tube that is inserted through the abdominal skin), which is removed a few weeks later.

Several months following the implant, repeat biopsies are performed to determine if any cancer remains. If cancer is still seen, the procedure can be repeated.

What patients are appropriate

The cryotherapy procedure itself is not much more involved than a repeat biopsy. Physically, most men can tolerate it.

What stages are appropriate

Theoretically, men with Stage A or B cancer would be the best candidates for cryo. Small Stage C cancers might be treated effectively. Patients with more advanced Stage C cancer are probably not good candidates, because cryo is unlikely to sterilize cancer that has spread outside of the prostate.

Cryotherapy is also used to treat men whose cancer has recurred within the prostate after radiation.

Side effects and complications

Very few meticulous reports regarding cryotherapy have been published. In the information available the likelihood of complications varies substantially, probably reflecting differences in skill, experience and the type of patients selected for treatment. The following numbers should be viewed skeptically.

Although cryo itself is a relatively minor procedure, the side effects have been substantial. Vague pain in the region of the prostate develops within several months in some patients.

The risk of urinary incontinence during the first year is approximately 2-10%. In experienced hands, there is perhaps a 0-5% risk of rectal damage, requiring surgical repair.

Most men are impotent afterwards, although some may regain potency within a year following treatment.

The results

As of 1996, there is minimal information regarding the effectiveness of cryo. The majority of men treated have negative repeat biopsies 3 months afterwards. Most still have some detectable PSA at that time. These results, which seem reproducible, are encouraging. The question that remains is what they mean in terms of eradication of cancer. Meaningful data regarding cancer eradication rates will probably not be available until the year 2000.

The near future

Cryo is still a very new procedure. There is tremendous controversy among doctors as to its merits. Some of the early results are encouraging. The likelihood of complications will probably continue to decrease, as more experienced is gained.

10

Comparing treatments

Determining the best treatment for prostate cancer can be difficult. Various legitimate treatment options are available, each with its pros and cons. In fact, a strong case can usually be made for more than one option. The best you can do, after reviewing the available information and considering the pros and cons of each treatment, is to make an educated choice as to which is best for you.

In considering the options, one must take several issues into account. Certainly the likelihood of cure is the first consideration. Also important is the impact that a treatment may have on your lifestyle.

Stage A and B cancers

Stage A and B cancers are the most curable—potentially curable with radiation or surgery. This chapter is focused on men with Stage A or B cancers, for which there is the most controversy regarding treatment.

Published reports favor surgery over radiation

Surgeons and radiation oncologists have been arguing for many years about whether surgery or radiation is more likely to cure men of prostate cancer. Most reports show better results with surgery compared to external radiation. However, historically, men treated with radiation have had more advanced cancers which are less likely to be cured regardless of what treatment is given. And while this bias in favor of surgery is not always clear in the medical reports, there is little doubt it exists.

External radiation compared to surgery

Only one trial has been conducted that directly compares surgery with external radiation. Performed in the U.S. Veteran's Administration hospitals in the 1960s, 97 patients were randomly assigned to be treated with surgery or radiation. The study showed that more patients were cured with surgery than with radiation. However, technical problems with the study caused the radiation community to dispute the results. Most problematic was that results of the radiation treatments were much inferior than what had been reported from other large medical centers. Whatever the reason for that, most radiation oncologists argue that the radiation results were not representative of what can be obtained today. If they were, it could be argued, the results of the VA trial would not have favored surgery so heavily.

Implants compared to external radiation or surgery

Results with implants, as of 1996, look comparable or somewhat better than those with external radiation. However, no scientific, rigorous trial has been performed to compare the two forms of radiation.

Results for Stage A or B cancers treated with implantation look similar or better than any results following prostatectomy. However, many surgeons argue that in the long run (greater than 10 years after treatment), there may be an advantage to surgery. This issue is unresolved. No scientifically run trials have been done that directly compare implants with surgery and no trials are planned at this time.

Fallacious arguments used to promote surgery

Doctors disagree as to how to best treat prostate cancer. Legitimate arguments can be made for and against each form of treatment. However, some unfounded arguments are made to advance one form of treatment over another. In particular, two fallacious arguments are commonly used to argue for the use of surgery over radiation. Common advice often given is to "just cut it out", implying that the simplest, surest treatment is to cut out the prostate. While this argument sounds valid, it is not. In up to 30 to 50% of men with Stage A or Stage B cancers, some cancer is left behind at the edge of the prostate.

A second argument often used to promote surgery asserts that if a man chooses radiation and it does not work, surgery afterwards will be more difficult. The implication is that if one has surgery first and it fails, a patient could have radiation as a salvage treatment. This argument, taken by itself, is true. However, it is not clear if the cure rate is any different whether radiation is given alone, or if it is used as salvage treatment after surgery fails. Patients who are not cured by surgery are probably the same ones who would not be cured with radiation, and vice versa. Someone who is not cured of prostate cancer with either form of treatment probably had more extensive cancer than was suggested by his pre-treatment studies. This is reflected by the fact that the cure rate the second time around with surgery or radiation is relatively low. Accordingly, it is probably not reasonable to choose one treatment type over the other based on the premise that another can be used if the first fails.

Summing it up

Surgery, external radiation and implants all have a legitimate place in the treatment of prostate cancer. Still unclear is which has the highest chance of curing cancer. To choose among treatments, one should consider the probable effectiveness, and the potential complications of each. *Table 10a* summarizes the major points to consider.

Table 10a

Treatment	*Pros*	*Cons*
Surgery	Best cure rate?	Big operation
		10% incontinence
		50%+ impotence
		Not for Stage C
		Disabled 2-6 wks
		Expensive
External radiation	Low complications	50%+ impotence
		Lower cure rate?
Implant	Easier than surgery	Relatively new
	Best cure rate?	
	Lower impotence	
Implant + External	Best for Stage C?	Relatively new
	Best for PSA >10?	Expensive
	Best for Gleason >7	

Cost

The cost of cancer treatment is high. Although cost has not been a major concern in choosing treatment in the past, it may become a factor in the future. The approximate cost of each type of treatment is listed in *Table 10b*. These numbers are rough estimates. The actual prices will vary by region of the country, and from hospital to hospital. Also, depending on how a procedure is performed, the cost could vary substantially. Furthermore, if complications occur, they could add substantially to the cost of treatment.

Table 10b

Treatment	_Approximate total cost_
Prostatectomy	$20,000
External radiation	$16,000
Implant alone	$10,000
Implant+external radiation	$25,000

11

Metastases and hormonal therapy

Prostate cancer is partially dependent on the presence of male hormones for its growth. Consequently, counteracting or depleting these male hormones will cause most prostate cancers to go into remission. Although hormonal treatment will put most prostate cancers into remission, doctors often disagree as to when the use of such therapy is indicated. The clearest indication for the use of hormone treatment is the presence of advanced, widespread, metastatic cancer. However, some physicians advocate using hormone treatment for Stage A or B cancers as well.

Metastases to lymph nodes versus metastases to bone

When cancer spreads away from a man's prostate, it goes to his lymph nodes around the prostate. With time, the cancer spreads from the lymph nodes to other parts of the body. Most often, it spreads to the bones. The cancer cells also circulate to other types of organs, but metastatic prostate cancer grows most readily inside bones.

Because prostate cancer cells are generally slow-growing, some men live for many years, even after cancer has spread to the lymph nodes or bones. But men with cancer only in the lymph nodes live longer than those whose cancer has spread to their bones. The chance of living five years after cancer has spread to the lymph nodes is approximately 80%. The probability of living five years after cancer has spread to the bones is about 20% (*Figure 10a*).

Unfortunately, men with cancer in the lymph nodes are probably not curable. But, having said that, some researchers believe a small percentage of men with cancer in the lymph nodes still can be cured by removal of their prostate and all the surrounding lymph nodes or by radiation to the lymph nodes. More likely, however, is that the few men who appear

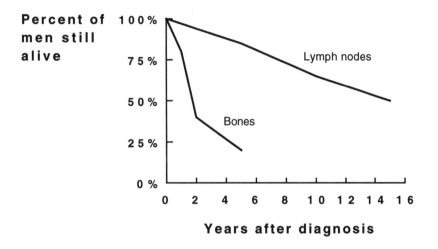

Figure 10a. Survival after diagnosis of cancer metastases in the lymph nodes versus in the bones.

cured after this treatment are those who have especially slow-growing cancers, and who would have lived many years even if they had not been treated.

Prostate cancer is partially dependent on male hormones

The growth of normal prostate cells and prostate cancer cells depends on the male hormones, testosterone and dihydrotestosterone. Consequently, if male hormones are removed from the body, most prostate cancers will shrink dramatically. Treatment that is intended to deplete the male hormones is termed "hormonal ablation."

Ways to deplete male hormones

CASTRATION (ORCHIECTOMY)

The idea of castration makes most men uncomfortable. But for those who can cope with the psychological implications, it is the simplest way to deplete males hormones, probably with less side effects than other methods.

The testicles produce nearly all the male hormones. Surgically removing the testicles, called castration or orchiectomy, eliminates 95% of the male hormones from the body. Castration is technically a minor, inexpensive operation, one not requiring overnight hospitalization or medication.

Side effects of castration are those that result from a loss of the hormones. About one-third of men have hot flashes, similar to those women experience with menopause, and most men lose their sexual desire and their ability to have erections.

FEMALE HORMONES

Another way to deplete male hormones is to receive female hormones. The brain detects the presence of female hormones and stops production of male hormones by the testicles. The most commonly used female hormone for this purpose is diethylstilbesterol (DES). The usual dose is one to three mg, once a day, by mouth.

Like castration, use of DES causes patients to experience hot flashes, loss of sexual desire and impotence. In addition to the side effects of castration, about one-third of men who take female hormones experience fluid retention and uncomfortable breast swelling. At higher doses than those used now, DES can cause blood clots and strokes.

PITUITARY INTERFERENCE

The pituitary gland, a small region on the underside of the brain, releases a hormone called gonadotropin. Gonadotropin circulates through the blood and signals the testicles to produce testosterone. In this way, the brain controls the amount of testosterone the testicles make.

In the 1980s, several drugs were developed to prevent the pituitary gland from signaling the testicles to produce male hormones. Such drugs include leuprolide (Lupron™) and gosorelin (Zoladex™), which are given to patients by monthly injection under the skin. Lupron™ or Zoladex™ are less likely to cause hot flashes, heart disease, or impotence than female hormones. Their primary disadvantage, however, is they require that patients undergo expensive monthly injections (costing approximately $350 per month).

ANTI-HORMONES (ANTI-ANDROGENS)

Approximately 95% of testosterone is made in the testicles. The remaining 5% is made in the adrenal glands (located just above the kidneys). This 5% of testosterone is not affected by castration, female hormones or pituitary interference, and even this small amount of testosterone may encourage the growth of a prostate cancer. To get the maximum benefit of hormone treatment, it is probably best to take a drug to stop the effect of testosterone produced by the adrenal glands.

Two such drugs are flutamide (Eulexen™) and bicalutaride (Casodex™). Both drugs prevent attachment of testosterone to prostate cells. Because they interfere directly with testosterone, they are called "anti-hor-mones." The medical term is "anti-androgens," derived from "androgen," a technical word for male hormones.

The added effect of anti-hormones, combined with other hormonal treatments, is probably small. However, it has shown some benefit, at least in men who have been castrated. According to several stud-ies, men who took anti-hormones, in addition to cas-tration or Lupron™/Zoladex™, lived several months longer than those who did not take anti-hormones. This effect is seen primarily in men with few metas-tases and who generally feel well at the start of treat-ment.

The primary side effect of flutamide is diarrhea, which affects about 10% of men. (The occurrence of diarrhea is lower with bicalutaride.) Liver damage is a small risk from taking flutamide, so that a blood test for liver enzymes should be checked every three months. Flutamide must be taken three times a day, for a cost of about $300-400 per month.

Comparing hormonal treatments

Several types of hormonal treatment are now available to men. While the newer drugs are not necessarily more effective, they usually have fewer side effects than female hormones. Several newer drugs will soon be available and may offer even more advantages. *Table 11a* summarizes the pros, cons and costs of each type of hormonal treatment.

Table 11a

Treatment	*Pros*	*Cons*	*Cost*
Castration	Easy	Psychologically difficult	$1500
Female hormones	Cheap	Hot flashes Fluid retention Heart problems	$30/month
Leupron™/ Zoladex™	Less menopausal effects Less impotence	Expensive	$350/month
Eulexen™/ Casodex™	Greater survival?	Diarrhea 10%	$350/month

Likelihood that hormonal therapy will work

Eighty percent of prostate cancers are sensitive to hormonal ablation, meaning that it will cause them to shrink substantially. Hormone treatment shrinks cancer within the prostate, as well as cancer that has metastasized. On average, the effect lasts two years, although in some men it can last much longer.

Does hormonal ablation treatment prolong life?

The beneficial effect of hormone therapy for treating prostate cancer is indisputable. However, there is considerable controversy as to whether it actually prolongs a patient's life. It seems sensible that any treatment which shrinks a cancer would prolong life, however, it is not clear whether this is truly the case.

After the effect of hormonal treatment wears off it appears that a patient's cancer begins to grow again and eventually reverts to what it would have been had the treatment never been given. If hormonal ablation is started again at a later time after they have stopped working, they usually do not work again.

For those men whose prostate cancer has advanced to the stage where it is causing problems, such as blockage of urine outflow or bone pain, hormonal treatment is usually the first choice of treatment. However, for patients whose prostate cancer has not progressed to that point, the use of hormone treatment is controversial, because these patients have no specific symptoms that need to be alleviated. For them, receiving treatment early will probably result in its ineffectiveness if used at a later time.

Large experimental trials were run in the United States Veteran's Administration hospitals in the 1960s, showing that hormonal ablation probably does not prolong survival in patients with Stage C prostate cancer. Some doctors, however, argue that previous trials do not apply to men with cancers at earlier stages. Men with smaller cancers, they argue, may be cured if treatment is started sooner, since they had less cancer at the outset. This argument is supported by data from the Mayo Clinic, which reported on men treated for prostate cancer with involvement of the lymph nodes. Men with tumors of low Gleason scores lived longer if they received hormonal treatment before any symptoms appeared. The Mayo studies, however, were not done in a strict, scientific fashion. Unforeseen reasons could have affected why some men did or did not receive hormonal treatment and this could explain why those who received hormonal therapy lived longer. The issue of whether treatment should be started sooner rather than later is still unresolved.

Chemotherapy

Chemotherapy refers to the use of toxic drugs to treat cancer. The drugs themselves can be thought of as poisons. Consequently, the chemicals are poisonous to all types of cells. However, some types of cancer are more sensitive to chemotherapy than normal cells. A sensitivity to relatively low doses of chemotherapy means that some cancer types can be eradicated by this method. Types of cancer that can usually be cured with chemotherapy include leukemias, testicle tumors, and lymphomas. Unfortunately, prostate cancers are not usually responsive to chemotherapy. Approximately 20% of prostate cancers will shrink with chemotherapy, but the shrinkage lasts only about two months. Unfortunately, there is little chance of being cured of prostate cancer with the chemotherapy drugs available as of 1996.

Some progress in combining different chemotherapy drugs has been made, resulting in higher probability that a patient's cancer will shrink. Considerable effort is being made in this area, and it is hoped that more effective drug combinations will become available. Because there is some chance that available chemotherapy can put prostate cancer in temporary remission, it is worth considering enrolling in an experimental trial of chemotherapy at a medical center. In general, it would be best to do so as part of legitimate research trial so that information from each patient's response to the drugs can be used to help determine better ways to use these drugs in the future.

12

Dealing with impotence

Sexual impotence is the most common complication of treatment for prostate cancer. It is caused by surgical or radiation damage to nerves and/or blood vessels that are normally responsible for filling the penis with blood to form an erection.

What is impotence

Impotence refers to the inability to have an erection, while the desire for sex is unchanged. Impotence due to radiation is usually permanent, and impotence lasting more than one year after prostatectomy is usually irreversible. Fortunately, there are a number of ways impotence can be corrected.

Loss of potency following treatment should not be attributed to psychological factors; it is usually due to the treatment. However, in some instances, potency can be diminished by psychological factors. A patient or his partner may fear that sex can either spread cancer to the partner, or somehow decrease the chances of being cured. Both notions are unfounded. If psychological issues may be interfering, a couple should consult a sex therapist.

How impotence may be corrected

ORAL DRUGS

Some oral drugs, including yohimbine, anti-depressants and vitamin E, may be effective treatment. While these drugs are not as effective as the mechanical measures described below, their side effects are usually minimal and they are worth trying.

PENILE RING

The simplest remedy for men with a partial loss of potency is to place an elastic constricting ring at the base of the penis after achieving as much of an erection as possible. The ring helps prevent blood outflow from the penis, thus helping to maintain an erection. This penile ring may be most effective for men who still have some ability to achieve an erection.

A ring should not be used for more than 30 minutes, to avoid bruising the penis. Only legitimate, commercial devices should be used.

VACUUM DEVICES

Vacuum devices are cylinders that fit around the penis. A hand, or electrically-operated pump creates a vacuum inside the tube to draw blood into the penis. Using this, it takes several minutes to develop an erection, at which time an elastic band is placed at the base of the penis to preserve the erection during intercourse.

Vacuum devices are usually effective, but can be somewhat cumbersome. Men should make sure to get adequate training in the proper technique by an experienced urologist.

SELF-INJECTION

Several drugs (papaverine, phentolamine, prostaglandins) can be injected directly into the base of the penis causing the blood vessels to widen, thus allowing more blood to flow into the penis and causing an erection. The dose of the drugs can be adjusted to allow an erection for about an hour. The needle is tiny and the injection is not considered painful. Approximately two-thirds of men can achieve a satisfactory erection with the injection method.

A complication that can arise from injection is some superficial scarring of the penile skin where the injections are given. Such scarring is usually minimal and of no particular consequence. Also, about 5% of men will develop a prolonged erection and need to go to a doctor's office or emergency room for an antidote injection.

Understandably, most men are not thrilled with the idea of using an injection. But in fact, self-injection is probably the most accepted way to obtain an erection, in those men willing to try it.

The drugs used for injections are widely available, but have not been approved by the FDA for treating impotence. The injection method, therefore, is technically considered experimental. This can cause difficulty with insurance re-imbursement for the cost of treatment.

PENILE IMPLANT

The surest way to restore the ability to have an erection is a plastic implant, permanently placed inside the penis. The device can have a semi-flexible rod inside, that can be repeatedly bent into the erectile versus normal position. Alternatively, an inflatable pump can be placed inside the patient's scrotum or above the base of his penis. The pump can be manually used to inflate the device when needed.

Implanted devices are usually effective but carry more risk of complications than other forms of treatment. The procedure required to place the device inside the penis destroys any remaining natural erection ability. There is a risk of infection and such infection might necessitate removal of the pump, especially in men with diabetes or bladder infections. If the device must be removed, scarring or shortening of the penis may occur afterwards. Additionally, there is approximately a 5% chance of mechanical difficulties with the devices, depending on the particular model used and the length of time it is left in place.

Summing it up

There are a variety of potentially effective treatments for impotence. It seems reasonable to start with the least drastic method (oral drugs), and try more involved methods if you are not satisfied.

Impotency treatments: Pros and cons

Method	*Pros*	*Cons*
Oral drugs	Easy	May be ineffective
Penile ring	Easy Fairly effective	Must be partially potent
Vacuum device	Effective	Somewhat cumbersome Some penile bruising
Self-injection	Effective	Injection required Penile scarring possible Prolonged erection possible
Implanted device	Effective	Risk of infection Expensive

13

Where to get help

If you understand most of the concepts in this book, you have a fairly good idea of the pros and cons of each form of treatment for prostate cancer. These concepts form the basis of what your doctors will discuss with you. Of course, one could quibble about the details, but the numbers presented here are generally accepted by the medical community. Chances are that you have already spoken to at least one doctor about your cancer, and what should be done about it. If something in this book contrasts sharply with something your doctors have told you, it would be wise to ask them about the discrepancy. If you are still having trouble deciding what to do, seek further advice.

One source, besides consulting more doctors, are the patient support groups. The people who work for them are generally knowledgeable and can give you advice from a patient's perspective. Additionally, they have often already gone through the medical system and can give you a realistic idea of what to expect, from a patient's perspective. Listed below are some of the support groups you might contact:

American Cancer Society
1599 Clifton Road
Atlanta, Georgia
800-ACS-2345

Make Today Count
800-432-2273

Man to Man (American Cancer Society)
800-432-2345

National Institute of Health
Cancer Information Service
800-4-CANCER

Patient Advocates for Advanced Cancer Treatments
(PAACT)
1143 Parmalee NW
Grand Rapids, MI 49504
616-453-1477

Prodigy On-line Support Group
Ron Koster, founder
75 Florence Street
Kingston, NY 12401-3017
914-338-8005
E-Mail: NWNG30A@PRODIGY.COM

Prostate Cancer Resource Network
P.O. Box 966
New Port Richey, Florida 34656
813-842-9758

US TOO Support Groups, Inc.
P.O. Box 7173
Oak Brook Terrace, Illinois 60181
800-80-US-TOO

Index

To order additional copies of
Prostate Cancer: A Non-surgical Perspective,
call toll free:
(800) 345-6665 (VISA/Mastercard).

Or send a check or money order for
$15.95 U.S. / $17.95 Canadian
plus $4.00 shipping and handling to:

SmartMedicine Press
407 New Concord Road
Canaan, NY 12060

Please allow 3-6 weeks for delivery when
ordering by mail.

New York State residents please add $1.60 sales tax.